TH

ENERGY

RESET

THE ENERGY RESET

LAURA & BARRY ASH

First published in 2023

ISBN 978-0-9956648-9-0

Book design: Laura and Barry Ash and Danny Lyle

Editing: Laura and Barry Ash

CONTENTS

FOREWORD

I met Loz and Baz through a serendipitous event in 2016, at a self-help/development course in London. In a room full of hundreds of people I was (at the time unexplainably) drawn to them. I told them how I was a Consultant Psychiatrist working in London, as well as a carer for my dad that had bowel cancer, and they in turn told me how they were health and fitness small-business owners from Folkestone in Kent. We then went on to bond over our love of cats and all things a bit "woo". We went on to share a couple of lunches and dinners and I thought that was that, but also knew there was something special about them. They genuinely listened and wanted to help.

We stayed in touch every now and again and I attended one of their Rock Solid events in the winter of that year. What I didn't know at the time was that Loz and Baz would become my saviours in years to come. In 2017 Loz and I were supposed to go to the advanced version of the course we did the year before. Closer to the time I couldn't go as my father had developed a second unrelated cancer so Loz attended on her own, and then had the beginnings of her "breakdown" during the course. I stayed in touch and learned more about Loz and Baz's background and what they did and how they used all experiences to learn and turn it into something positive. Loz became a mental health spokesperson for the time to change campaign, and Baz overcame his dyslexia and fear of public speaking by doing a full on talk to a group of 200 people.

Fast forward to 2020-21, which was not only the time of Covid-19, but also the time they broke the news to me, that what I had was classic burnout. All of a sudden, I had an explanation and a name for what I was experiencing: I was constantly worn-out; I was existing rather than living; becoming more withdrawn; feeling low; and my "can-do" attitude had turned into a "I really can't be bothered" attitude. I was not only disappointed in myself but also shocked that I hadn't recognised it in myself or wanted to (if I'm honest). After much reflection, my question was "now what?"

As usual, Loz and Baz's timing was perfect, there was a "free energy-management" workshop that they were running for an hour a day, for a couple of days. My God was this an eye-opener as to how much I had let my true self go. This eventually led to me signing up to do their 12-month "Energised Leadership" course. This helped me step-by-step to go back to the basics of the 6 pillars and go through a "reset": accepting and acknowledging what was going on, creating awareness, taking some intentional action, and then finally assess and adjust the plan to my needs.

Now I'm not saying that I am "cured" of burnout but I can confidently say I feel like the enthusiastic person I was and now am. Amazingly despite being burnt-out I became a Fellow of the Royal College of Psychiatrists' and now put my own self-care above most things (not all), all thanks to Loz and Baz's guidance and my will to learn. This book will help you do the same, as a step-by-step guide of recognising burnout and more importantly the steps you can take to help yourself.

If there was any time the nation needed help to deal with burnout, this is the time, and Loz and Baz give you the weapons you need to beat it. They use their own lived experiences to help you. PLEASE take that help.

Dr Khadijah Hussain, BSc (Hons), MBBS, FRCPsych and human-being that knows how to be down, but definitely NOT OUT!

INTRODUCTION

Welcome! We're Loz and Baz and we want to thank you for picking up our book.

We've learned so much, personally and professionally, over the years and we wanted to share it with you. We've used the strategies and tools in this book for ourselves and our clients for many years to get ourselves back into credit in our 'energy bank account'.

We're writing this book in the midst of the pandemic and it will be no surprise to you that people all over the world are exhausted and mental health challenges are at an all-time high. There couldn't be a better time to share our tried and tested energy reset programme with you.

No matter where you are at right now, no matter how low or fatigued, this will help you look differently at your energy and how it works. It will help – we promise!

WHO ARE WE?

First, we should tell you a bit about us and what inspired us to write this book. We'll keep it brief because we want to get on to telling you about the transformation you can make happen in your life.

Baz has been involved in fitness and health for 25 years. He was a fitness instructor, then a personal trainer. He made the big decision to leave that career behind and join the Prison Service. He walked those landings for 3 years but never lost his burning desire for health and fitness. In Prison Services officers are able to specialise so it gave him a chance to use his experience to teach prisoners about physical education. More than that he was able to help them to become personal trainers, fitness instructors and sports therapists which gave them career and job options once they left prison, as well as their own healthier lifestyle. He left the prison service after 10 years and set up Rock Solid with Loz.

Loz's background is definitely not in fitness. She freely admits that she didn't enjoy fitness related activities until she joined the police force. She's a former police and counter terrorism officer. At 33 years old she was medically retired from the force because of a diagnosis of bipolar (bipolar affective disorder) and OCD (obsessive compulsive disorder). She was completely convinced that no-one would give her a job because of her health issues, so setting up Rock Solid Health was a no-brainer

Rock Solid Health, which is based in Kent, is our business that was set up initially to help people transform their bodies back in 2013.

However, we soon realised that was only one piece of the puzzle. Since then it has evolved and we now work with clients globally, and corporate organsiations.

We offer strategies and programs to organisations to help the health and well-being of their staff.

We show our 1-2-1 clients how to restore their health, get back thier energy, during or post burnout, enabling them to live a fulfilled live creating more time to do the things they love through our 6 pillars of health and well-being (which you will find out more about during this book)

WHY DID WE WRITE THIS BOOK?

We've learned so much through our professional and personal experience. Working through Loz's diagnosis, managing her energy and her subsequent breakdown in 2017, which you will learn more about soon, has given us so much incredibly valuable experience and knowledge that we felt it would be criminal not to share it and show others that things can get better and how to make that happen.

A lot of the learning we've gained in this area comes out of what we have done for ourselves and how we've looked after ourselves and each other. As we said earlier, we started Rock Solid because Loz suffered an epic breakdown through burnout.

We were both working all hours of the day and night. Loz was well and truly burning the candle at both ends. The other critical factor was that she hadn't identified a success path so she could measure how far she'd come. In 2017 she literally went 'bang' overnight and was so flattened by it she could only do colouring in. We faced almost losing our business.

At that point, we said, right, this is where we put our stake in the ground. We took our professional and personal experiences to determine what the critical parts of the process to getting back on track, not being burned out and putting our energy in credit are, to ensure we manage our energy effectively and ensure longevity, resilience and a great quality of life. We've all seen the fitness industry fail people time and time again. We think that's because all factors of health need to be taken into account and all of our extensive experience has been put into our Energy Reset Programme, which we're sharing with you in this book. Our five-step process has worked for so many of our clients and we want to share it with more people than we can possibly get to one to one. We really want people to benefit from this, to get themselves out of burn-out in a sustainable way and have the life they really want. There are so many of you out there who've experienced some version of what Loz has been through.

We share our own stories in the book so that you can see how we've used them to change our own lives, and to put our knowledge and experience into transforming our own energy. We practice what we preach. You'll see these stories throughout the book in text boxes.

WHICH BRINGS US ON TO, WHO IS GOING TO GET THE MOST OUT OF THIS BOOK

You are in the right place to get the value from our experience if you're already experiencing symptoms like exhaustion or a lack of interest in things that would usually stoke your passions. This book is for people who want to manage their energy in a sustainable way to avoid burn-out and the vast range of symptoms it brings with it, and for those who want to avoid it by not 'overdrawing' their energy account.

If feeling healthier and more resilient isn't motivation enough, then think about this. You've got into what you do because you love it. We fall out of love with what we do when our energy is overdrawn. What drives us is for you to feel that passion again so you can get your enthusiasm and energy back. You'll start enjoying life and having the abundance of what you want out of this life. Sounds great, doesn't it?

Dolly Parton has a fantastic quote which sums up what you will get from this book

---

"Don't get so busy making a living that you FORGET to make a life"

It's truly brilliant and sums up how much we need to ensure that we don't just focus on our work life which is important BUT also to create a fulfilling life experience because you are only here once and you're not meant to be a workhorse.

You're going to learn more about how to manage your energy looking at how much energy you have and how you expend it during the day.

You're also in the right place if you manage a team or business, and you want to help your staff proactively manage their energy. Your team is your number one resource and your organisation is only as resilient as they are. We need to stop seeing resilience as 'persistence and tenacity'. That stuff is great but what if your team managed their energy so well that they didn't need to work long hours, drink loads of caffeine or binge on chocolate to be at their most productive and creative?

This book is going to take you through the entire Energy Reset Programme. We've also added in some workbook space for you to record your thoughts and decisions on your journey through the programme.

Before we start there is something you need to agree to if you want to really see the transformational changes that are available to you from what we've got to share.

Make a pact with yourself.

THIS IS A JUDGEMENT FREE ZONE

We are not going to judge ourselves. Do yourself a favour and free yourself from judgement during this. We're going to be taking an honest look at some of the things we do and how we feel. The more honest you are the more you'll get out of it. Any change worth making needs to start with a frank look, assessment and acknowledgement, of where you're at. It doesn't matter where you are at right now. The chances are that you and everyone you know will find themselves experiencing some or even all of what we talk about in these next 6 chapters. What matters is what you're going to do about it.

We asked others who had been through the Energy Reset Program what their experience was and what they got from it

We wanted to share that here for you know what to expect in the coming pages

"I did it because I was feeling overwhelmed with my workload and felt that I would never get through it - it just felt like a massive mountain to climb! I also realised that I was burnt out and this meant that I had a negative attitude towards my work; this made it really hard to motivate myself to do stuff and it sucked all the job satisfaction that I used to get from my work right out! Realising that cynicism was a symptom of burnout helped to me to stop criticising myself for feeling that way and the stuff about energy and time really got me thinking about how I use these, and to develop strategies to use them for greater effect" - Pam

"During 2020, as Laura put it, I went BANG. I had to start my business from scratch due to leaving the gym I previously worked from. I was very overwhelmed and I was burning the candle at both ends but not feeling like I was achieving anything at the end of each day. I put enormous pressures on myself and it caught up with me.

Doing the energy reset with Loz and Baz just seemed to land on my lap at the right time. I was thinking of beginning work again but didn't know how I would manage without going BANG again. The energy reset course gave me the space and permission to address what was actually going on and what factors led to burn out. I think stand out moment for me was "you have a duty of care to yourself" for your clients, friends, family and business.

I had never thought of it like that. Also the analogy that energy= money.... I soon discovered I wasted a lot of "money" not refilling my cup and procrastinating in fear I wouldn't succeed.

I couldn't recommend this course enough, it was just what I needed to reset my energy and my outlook on how I manage my day. I already feel more in control and doing things with purpose that will drive me forward instead of on tail spin. Thankyou thank you thank you!" - Steffie

"In the last year I have been struggling with how to keep myself moving and motivated, especially with everything the world is going through right now! The training helped be to refocus on what is most important, being authentic to myself and making sure to care for myself!" - Melissa

"I learned that I need to look after myself in order to provide effective energy in the workplace. I realised that I need to fill up my own cup in order to pour energy effectively to colleagues and students. It has brought the importance of looking after myself to the fore. It is easy to plough all your energy into work and head for burnout. This course made me take stock and audit the use of my time and energy. It was a brilliant course full of so much wonderful information that can be put into practice. Thank you Laura and Barry....you are both amazing" - Belinda

"By putting Into practice what I learned from this program will not only change your working life by giving you the tools to improve your working life but it also benefits outside work as I am not frazzled by end of the week and not thinking of work all the time as when I'm not at work that is my time! This I feel makes me more productive at work and helps me to give my clients with a better service" - Lorraine

"Laura and Barry put so much into everything they do. They are approachable and really motivating. The training definitely opened my eyes to new ways of thinking about myself, my business and my future. It was very thought provoking. I can highly recommend" Katie

"For me this was an eye opener. I was given examples of how burn out can affect you mentally, physically and I was a lot of these always negative. Not looking after my basic needs all had a knock on affect. I went to bed late one night and the next day I was irritable, was making bad food/drink choices didn't want to do anything. A complete lack of motivation. But I recognised that for what it was and the following night I was in bed on time. It's about stepping back and looking at why am I like this? And being non judgemental. I would always work whilst eating at my desk now I go into the staff room. Just that little time away made me feel better. Time to reset my mind" Terry-Ann

CHAPTER ONE

Our story

If you change the way you look at things, the things you look at change

Dr Wayne Dyer

It's hard to believe that when we first started, we were doing simple beauty transformations. It was all about the physical body and how it looked. That's what we were into and we thought everyone wanted to make their exteriors look the best they could.

We started to notice that you can look great on the outside but that doesn't mean that you've made permanent changes on the inside. We were really helping people by building their confidence but we really wanted to change people's lives. So, we started down a path of not just working on people's bodies but transforming their lives through working on their minds and behaviours as well.

We started to realise this through our bodybuilding experience. We'd both done three bodybuilding competitions and this was Baz's moment of clarity.

'I had it in my head that I needed to have the experience of a a particular competition with a men's bodybuilding magazine.

It was my first time on stage and I spent six months preparing for this one competition. I had an expectation that when I got on stage, I would feel something mega.

As that light shone down on me, I was so sure that I would suddenly see myself as a different, "new" me. We've all seen those ads about body transformations – we're promised a perfect body, world class confidence and limitless energy.

I got on stage, hit my first post, with that light shining directly on me. I waited for the promised feeling, the 'mega me'. What I realised was that I was still Baz. I was still exactly the same person. I'm having exactly the same voice and exactly the same internal conversation. I was ripped from my toenails to my hair follicles. My body looked totally different.

That's when the penny drops. I can see clearly for the first time that it's the industry that needs to change – it needs an almighty kick in the ass. Because ultimately, it's not about the physical. It's not about how your body looks. It's not about the aesthetics. It's all about how we feel as human beings. Nothing on the outside is going to change what's happening on the inside.' **Baz**

'In 2016 and we were struggling in the business. Every business goes through it – trying to find our feet. We were trying to work out what our mission and message were and to identify our ideal client. We were working all of the hours that God sent.

At the time we had a coach called Mark Whitehand and he kept saying to me "Loz you really need to manage your energy" I was agreeing with him but not really paying attention (sorry Mark).

Until it knocked me flat on my face in 2017. 2017 was such a busy year for us. We had an uncomfortable feeling that we weren't being our true, authentic selves. In trying to make the business work, we'd become more focussed on money than on what our clients needed. It had crept up on us.

Changing our clients' lives was our mission but our days felt like they'd become about bringing in an income. So, we decided to pivot the business to bring it back on track with our mission. The outcome of getting into business is a good income, in the same way that the output of looking after ourselves is weight loss or muscle gain, but we wanted to refocus on our purpose and let the income become a by-product of us focusing on what really mattered to us – health!

We hadn't realised just how much we'd taken on. We were burning the candle at both ends – going into London for meetings, staying up late to get work finished and just doing far too much. As happens so often with business-people we were suffering from comparisonitis and seeing so many people around us doing so well, and feeling like we were just not measuring up. That was a vicious cycle because it just meant we tried to work harder. There is a lot of toxic positivity around running a business. You'll all have seen the social posts telling you to 'go hard or go home' which just pushed us into doing more and more. There was no way our business was going to fail because we weren't 'going hard'. Looking back now. we can see that during May, June and July of 2017 something was brewing. The signs were there right in front of us. We were doing what we could see our clients doing, trying to set up their own businesses.

It is easy to ignore the signs when the world of social media is telling you that you are only a winner if you are driving yourself and that working hard is 'morally good'. It's not so long ago that going to bed early or sleeping later was seen as laziness and a lack of ambition.

I admit that I was being reckless with my mental health. I recognise now that I was in full blown mania and ignoring it because I was spiralling. I know anyone who has been there will recognise when you have these manic episodes your head gets so busy and full. The only comparison I can give is that it's like having someone sing happy birthday, counting to ten, thinking about your to-do list and reciting the alphabet all at the same time, on repeat.

I just couldn't stop the relentless noise in my head. It was literally midnight on 25th July 2017 and I went bang! By bang I mean I couldn't sleep. I burst into uncontrollable crying until about four in the morning. I still couldn't see that anything was wrong. Baz and our PA, Toni, had to take the reins.

Baz called the crisis team and got me to speak to a nurse. They told me that I really did need some help. I had one of the biggest breakdowns since I'd left the police in 2013. It wasn't just my mental health – my physical and emotional health was at an all-time low.

I'd hit the peak of burn-out. I couldn't dress myself or even make a cup of tea. The only thing I could do was to colour-in. That all happened on Saturday and by Wednesday I sat back at my desk but I burst into tears because even checking my emails was too overwhelming.

We nearly lost the business because I couldn't work. I'd been so reckless and irresponsible with my mental health and hadn't managed my energy.' **Loz**

After that we took a stand and used our experiences, particularly those above, and created the 6 pillars. So much of it was what we'd used to help Loz get her health back, so we knew they worked.

As soon as we started acting on these 6 pillars our health started to come back. The human body, mind and spirit are amazing tools. If we look after them then they will do anything we need them to do. If we abuse it or overuse them, they will let us know. We believe, in part, that is what burn-out is. If we start misusing the 6 pillars and overwhelming our mental, emotional, physical and spiritual body then they will kick back. If we don't listen to the early signs then we will burn out. If we really ignore it then we will experience a bang, as we call it.

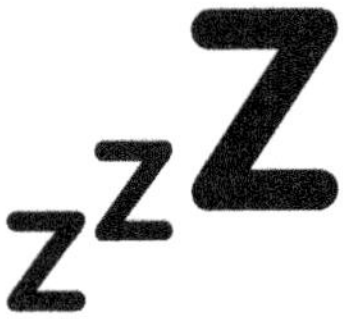

SLEEP

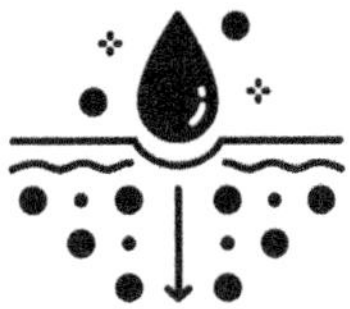

HYDRATION

NOURISHMENT

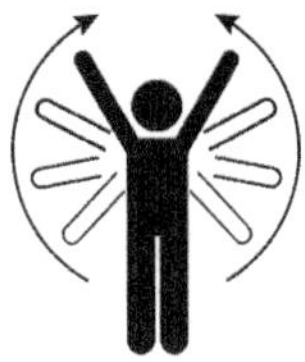

MOVEMENT

THOUGHT MANAGEMENT

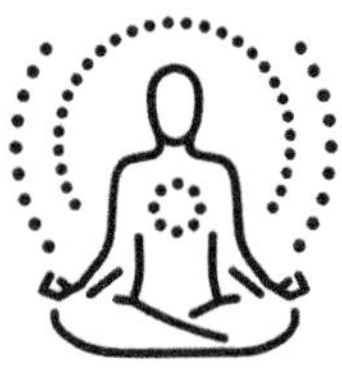

DESTRESSMETIME

We've taken time over the past 18 months of the pandemic to really look at what our skills and abilities are. We run a successful business and manage a very serious and chronic mental health condition which has acute episodes. It's not just bipolar which, in comparison to the OCD, is easy. We feel strongly that it would be criminal for us not to take this knowledge and experience and share with other people, how to manage their energy for themselves, and avoid the 'big bang'.

As we get back to whatever the world's new normal will be, there will be new challenges on top of the old ones. We have worked in high pressure jobs and run a successful business that actually grew in the pandemic. We've taken all our expertise, knowledge and passion and created the Energy Reset and Energised Leadership Programmes.

Business owners are the most likely group to kick start our ailing economies and so the whole world is going to need people like you to be in tip top condition.

Reduced income, pivoting our businesses, uncertainty, home schooling and health have all been competing for our attention. That has meant we've been working too many hours, doubling up teaching our kids and taking less holidays and a lot of us are at breaking point. It's harder when we can't see the end in sight in this unprecedented situation, which brings stress of its own.

Our NHS is on its knees and its staff are suffering due to overstretched resources and losing patients and colleagues to this dreadful virus, while at the same time having had to spend significant time away from their own loved ones to avoid infecting them.

The fact is that so many of us are already in burn-out. Because it creeps up on us, many of us won't see it until it becomes critical. For that reason, we want this information in the public domain so you can use it to see where you are at right now and what simple, practical things you can do to manage your energy and avoid going bang.

WHY ENERGY RESET?

It's true that we work in one of the biggest industries in the world. The fitness industry is worth upwards of £35billion.

However, we've all seen the fitness industry fail people time and time again. We think that's because all factors of health need to be taken into account and all of our extensive experience has been put into our Energy Reset Programme which we're sharing with you in this book. Our five-step process has worked for so many of our clients and as we said before – we really want to help as many people as possible. There are so many of you out there who've experienced some version of what Loz has been through.

WE WROTE THIS BOOK DURING THE PANDEMIC BECAUSE...

Over lockdown we've realised just how many business owners, entrepreneurs, corporate types, executives and professionals are on the edge of burn-out or have already gone bang. It's so important that you manage your energy because you are the backbone to this nation, to this world. You're the ones who are going to get this economy running again. Sharing this information is important to all of us.

CHAPTER TWO

What is burnout?

Burnout happens
when you avoid being
human for too long

Sam Kean

Before we get started on managing your energy, we want to share a couple of the terms and definitions we use in the book, to make sure we're all on the same page. There's no point sharing all this knowledge and experience if we're talking about different things.

In this chapter we're going to talk about burnout:

- *the definition of what is it?*
- *current research*
- *the three dimensions of burn-out*
- *energy and what it means in relation to burnout*

Then we'll take you through our six pillars of health and well-being so that you have all you need to follow what we're talking about.

WHAT IS BURN-OUT?

There are not many of us who haven't heard of 'burn-out' but have you ever really thought about what it means?

What do you think it is?

What does it mean to you?

People use it a lot but what actually is it?

Have you ever experienced burn-out? What does it feel like?

Take a few minutes before you move on to consider what it means to you. What does it look and feel like for you? You can write down your thoughts here.

It's definitely not a term that should be used loosely or freely. We have to be very careful about the labels that we use especially when we use them on ourselves.

Sometimes by labelling ourselves, we can DISable ourselves.

The words we use project into the energy around us and, as so many of us know, what we 'put out there' is so often what we get back.

Let's look at a couple of definitions. The WHO (World Health Organisation) is the specialist health part of the United Nations (U.N.) set up to address international public health. They say:

> 'Burn-out is a syndrome conceptualized as resulting from chronic workplace stress that has not been successfully managed. It is characterized by three dimensions:
> - feelings of energy depletion or exhaustion.
> - increased mental distance from one's job, or feelings of negativism or cynicism related to one's job; and
> - reduced professional efficacy.'[1]

The Cambridge Dictionary definition says:

> '...the state of having no energy or enthusiasm because of working too hard" or "extreme tiredness or a feeling of not being able to work any more, caused by working too hard.'[2]

So, what do these definitions have in common? Both are about working too hard and are saying, simply, that you're putting too much out and not putting enough in.

We know for us, we were working at all hours, going to meetings in London and trying to squeeze in some fun things like concerts. It was a crazy time. You are probably doing the same – if you're business owners or executives you're probably pushing yourself all of the time because you want those results. You've got that drive. But at some point, your drive runs out when your energy does.

If you're like us you are a high achiever so you want to do a good job. You're passionate and driven. But there is a fine line between being passionate and then falling over the edge into apathy (not feeling anything, or feeling indifferent) and exhaustion.

3 DIMENSIONS OF BURN-OUT

We found some great research on burn-out, which we felt illustrated its impact really well and fit with our methods and the 6 pillars of health and well-being.

3 Dimensions of Burn Out

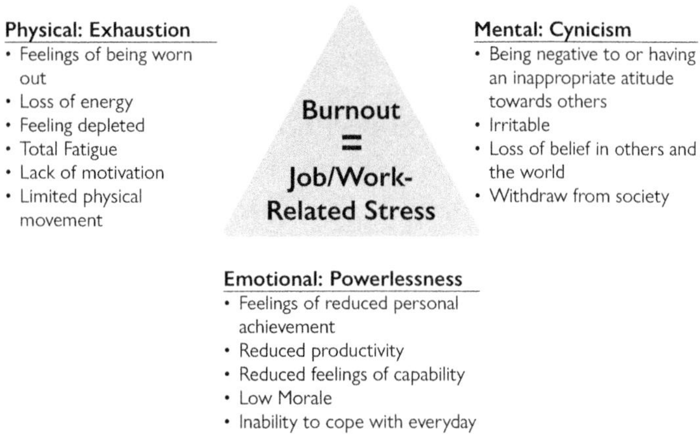

In 2016 *World Psychiatry* reported on a study by the Psychiatry Department of Berkeley and the Centre for Organizational Research and Development at Arcadia University. It looked specifically at the experience of burn-out.

It was really interesting and considered how to get people back into the workplace from a perspective of using psychiatry. We picked up on it and thought there was something compelling in this study that resonated with us and was consistent with our 6 pillars.

As you read more about the three dimensions of burn out perhaps you can think about which feel like you right now. It could help give you a real sense of where you're at. You might find you fall more into one dimension than another, or that you recognise yourself in all three.

We've taken this study and built on it by pairing exhaustion with physical burn-out, cynicism with mental burn-out and powerlessness with emotional burn-out. We've done this so you can identify and perhaps recognise some of the physical, mental and emotional symptoms and the way they make people feel. We have also taken it further and linked each of these three dimensions of burn-out with our six pillars.

Pillar 1(sleep), Pillar 2 (water), Pillar 3 (nourishment) and Pillar 4 (movement) match up with the exhaustion/physical dimension. Pillar 5 (thought management) matches up with the cynicism/mental dimension and Pillar 6 (DeStressMeTime) with the powerlessness/emotional dimension. You will see how they link naturally together as you go through each of the steps in the book.

EXHAUSTION/PHYSICAL

Let's look at the first dimension as exhaustion. The study defined the following as symptoms:

- *the feeling of being worn out*
- *the loss of energy*
- *feeling depleted*
- *total fatigue*
- *lack of motivation*
- *limited physical movement*

However, we've taken it further to identify what some of the actual physical symptoms of exhaustion look and feel like, from our own experience, personally and professionally, working with energy management. You might find you're:

- *doing little or no exercise*
- *not bothered to prepare food*
- *waking up tired*
- *having regular headaches*
- *always reaching for caffeine*
- *always reaching for high sugar foods*
- *gaining weight*

When we think about this dimension from an energy perspective it feels like giving up or wanting to give up. It feels very flat.

Have a think about some of these actions you might be doing and expand on them a little to see if you relate to them.

- ☐ *Are you opting for 'easy' or quick food instead of having the energy to make nutritious meals.*
- ☐ *Are you reaching for the high stimulant foods to 'fuel' you through the day.*

- [ ] *Are you finding that by doing some of these things you're putting on weight.*
- [ ] *Headaches can be a big one. If we're waking up with headaches or getting a lot of them during the day, we won't necessarily connect them with burn out or exhaustion.*

If you're fatigued your muscles can start tensing up and that can cause headaches.

Have you been experiencing any of these symptoms over recent weeks or months?

Which ones stick out for you?

You can record your thoughts here or even put a tick alongside those that feel like you right now.

____

____

____

____

____

POWERLESSNESS/EMOTIONAL

The next set of symptoms from the study are about powerlessness:

- *feelings of reduced personal achievement*
- *reduced productivity*
- *reduced feelings of capability*
- *low morale*
- *inability to cope with every day*

We looked at more of the emotional symptoms or indicators that you might be experiencing powerlessness as the study defined it. So, what might this look like for you on an everyday basis?

- *Emotional outbursts*
- *Never getting the 'to-do' list done*
- *Always putting off tasks*
- *Unable to concentrate*
- *Brain fog*
- *Flitting from job to job without completing the first one*
- *Questioning your destiny*
- *Looking for jobs (Especially Business Owners/Self Employed)*
- *Scrolling and comparing*

If you were to see this as an energy in your body it feels very much like it's deep in the pit of your stomach, a black oozy nauseous feeling. A very low energy that feels hopeless and immovable.

You might want to ask yourself these questions:

☐ *Are you struggling with controlling your emotions?*
☐ *Are you putting off tasks every day?*

- ☐ *Is your concentration rubbish and are you having trouble focussing on your work?*
- ☐ *Are you moving from job to job or task to task and questioning who you are and what you're meant to be doing with your life?*
- ☐ *Are you a business owner or self-employed person who has decided to look for a job?*
- ☐ *Are you endlessly engaged in the dreaded scroll or worse, are you comparing others' lives with yours?*
- ☐ *Are you asking yourself what others are doing that you're not doing? Are you comparing yourself with others?*
- ☐ *You might know you feel like this but how is it showing up for you in your life? What is the symptom? How many of those do you recognise that are happening for you right now?*

CYNICISM/MENTAL

The study showed their definition of cynicism featured the following:

- *Being negative or having an inappropriate attitude towards others*
- *Irritable*
- *Loss of belief of others and the world*
- *Withdrawl from society*

We see this as the mental/psychological side of burn-out. So how might this be showing up in your lives then?

- *Being over judgemental*
- *Angry outbursts*
- *Isolating self/choosing to stay indoors/can't be bothered going out*
- *Fighting with loved ones and friends*
- *Chest palpitations*
- *Seeing the bad in everyone*
- *Being overly negative*
- *Being sceptical/paranoid*

Cynicism is a tough one. None of us like to see ourselves as the 'Debbie Downer', or a 'Negative Nelly' or even just a plain old grump in people's lives. We would hate others to see us as the negative person in their world. But everyone has these times in their lives where they find it hard to get out of the funk they are in. Over the pandemic it has been hard not to feel downbeat about the state the world is in and the selfishness and ignorance evident. However, recognising this state in ourselves and accepting that we are experiencing it is critical to fixing it. This can feel like looking at the shadow side of ourselves and while we may not want to see it, try not to judge yourself for feeling like this, the chances are that it's a sign of burn-out.

When we look at this dimension from an energy point of view it feels tense, angry, low, negative or snappy energy. When we picture these in our minds it seems very sharp, very pointy or a heavy, flat, sad energy.

- ☐ *You could find yourself being overly judgemental with others but also with yourself. Are you judging others and yourself too harshly?*
- ☐ *You might be flying off the hook for what doesn't seem to be a good enough reason. Are you staying at home and isolating yourself from other people or having arguments with people you love for no reason at all?*
- ☐ *You could even be experiencing heart palpitations. Are you having physical symptoms like palpitations?*
- ☐ *You may only see the negative in your life and what you see seems to reinforce that making you even more negative. Are you feeling like it's hard to see things in your life from a positive perspective right now?*

When you look at these, which ones can you recognise? You may even find you can see many or all of these symptoms in your life, or a few ticks in each section. Remember that you are in a non-judgemental space here so you are not allowed to beat yourself up because of anything you recognise here.

STOP AND TAKE A DEEP BREATH

We'd be very, very surprised if any of you didn't see yourself somewhere in these symptoms.

Stop and take a deep breath at this point because that might have felt like a big slap in the face realising how many boxes you've ticked.

You don't need to worry about whatever you've identified here, or how many boxes you've ticked. As you read through this book you'll see that there are some very simple, sustainable strategies and tools to fix what you're seeing now.

STIGMA

Let's talk about the elephant in the room. There are a lot of people who say they don't believe in burn-out. They don't believe in mental health conditions. There are people who see not sleeping as some sort of weird badge of honour. Or they have a view that to be a winner you need to get up at some ungodly hour in the morning. You know, that whole 'you snooze, you lose', or 'you can sleep when you're dead' crowd. These are the people who see burn-out as some sort of weakness. The fact that it's only those who overwork who reach it eludes them. They'll ignore it until they've crashed and burned themselves and then like Loz they'll realise how crazy they've been, not looking after themselves and managing their energy better.

There is so much value in enjoying the journey rather than rushing full speed ahead towards a destination

---

We need to experience life every single day and have gratitude for what happens.

We've spoken to and worked with so many people in different sectors. Solicitors, for example, have told me about their colleagues and said that they would laugh in their face if anyone tried to talk to them about stress or burn-out. It doesn't exist because they don't have time for it. You see this is the way they behave at work and about work. There's a real sense of having to be available all of the time. If someone emails them at 10pm they need to be there to reply to it. Yet they'll still expect to be at their desk working by 9am. We rate those people who have been in since 7.30am and are still at their desks 12 hours later. This, apparently, shows dedication to the firm. But it doesn't value people's wellbeing. It's all about the company and their income and productivity and maximising both. They don't care about the welfare of their staff.

Corporates need to start investing in their team and their team's health and wellbeing. If they don't, their productivity and profits will go down. An organisation is only as strong as its greatest resources – their staff. If they don't look after them then their business will go down the pan. We've seen so much about resilience throughout the pandemic but a company is only as resilient as its team. If you aren't looking after them then your business won't perform at its best.

We spoke to a lady recently who worked for a company we'd approached to help them with some burn-out training. They told us they had that already. When we asked her what initiatives the company had invested in for the staff she said that they left a letter on the wall directing staff to a phone number if they were struggling right now. Not exactly robust or proactive.

It's a token gesture and will be just as effective. That company is clearly not taking its team's wellbeing seriously. Businesses are the same. We've all heard the language and it's all around 'hustling' 'being a winner' 'go hard or go home' – this is all telling us that if we're not working every hour of the day then we will never 'be a winner'. Yet that all feels like us have to force ourselves. Pushing ourselves beyond our sustainable limits to achieve more and more with our time and energy. Forcing ourselves is not the answer. If you're having to 'force' yourself then you're probably already struggling with burn-out. Businesses, like people, need everything to operate as well as it can – to look after your business, you need to look after yourself.

This is a two way street. Employees need to take responsibility for their own health and wellbeing, and not to push themselves beyond their limits. Companies and organisations must adopt a culture to support their staff, in real and practical ways.

That is why this book is so important to you, as an individual, so you can start to take action and responsibility for your health and have your employer back you up on these actions and practices.

There needs to be an open, two way conversation about boundaries, workloads and deadlines within the organisation. For this to work, change needs to start from the top and filter down, and it needs to be about actions, not just words.

Perhaps you could pop a copy of this book on your boss's desk WINK!

It's so important for us to be talking about burn-out right now because so many people are feeling this way. If the organisations and employers you work for aren't talking about it and acknowledging it then the chances are that you think you are the problem, that there is something wrong with you. There is nothing wrong with you. It's just that you've worked too hard and not balanced your other needs alongside your work. People are often fobbed off with anxiety and depression when they talk about it. They may have anxiety or depression but they are symptoms not the cause. The cause is very likely to be burn-out.

Our culture often has a lot to do with our high expectations of ourselves. We often compare ourselves to our mums and dads and what they achieved. They may have brought up five kids and so many of us wonder why we can't handle what they seemed to do so easily. We compare ourselves to them and find ourselves coming up short. Yes, your mum probably did run a household with five kids and that's a big job but she wouldn't necessarily have had to run a business or a career alongside that. Social media means that we constantly have comparisons about what other people are achieving in their lives and we feel like we don't measure up. Be aware that under those shiny profiles most of those people are probably feeling exactly the same way you are. And if you speak to your mum and dad, you'll probably find that they really struggled to get everything done, just as you are.

We are just so available now, thanks to technology. Some of it is so positive – the easier access and the instant capacity to connect. However, there is a huge downside. We are always so available and this has brought with it such a lot of expectations. In your parents' generation, so many had to wait for the postman to deliver documents. Phones were expensive and not always readily available. Very few had global businesses where they worked with people across a range of time zones, yet that is standard even for the smallest of businesses these days. Our phones, emails and social media ping with constant messages, constant calls on our time and getting away from that feels difficult and sometimes makes us feel guilty.

People in other centuries had different stresses and threats but if you read about some indigenous societies, they would work for as long as it took for them to hunt, gather and protect their tribe. That could be ten or fifteen hours in a week. Of course, their threats were very likely to be predators.

Our mental stress these days is huge. We often work at such a level of stress that we don't even notice it until we go on holidays or spend time in an environment where they don't do that. It's so much more prevalent in our society because we are constantly comparing ourselves and feeling like we are in a competition with others for money or clients. We don't want to lose our jobs or our careers so we feel under pressure to work harder to ensure that doesn't happen.

If you're reading this and you are a leader or a manager then you've got to think about the fact that you set the example for your team. We have a client who says that she feels she needs to email at 10pm at night because her colleagues and employees are. We said to her – but you are the leader. They are taking their steer from you. If you start leading by example and shutting your laptop at 6pm and putting an out of hours on saying you will respond when you are back in the office at 9am, then your team will see that and know that that is the new normal. You set the bar for them. If they see you at your desk replying to emails at 10pm then they will feel like they have to do that as well because we are a nation of people pleasers and we want to be seen to be doing 'the right thing'. So, if you are in that kind of position then you are a role model. They are looking up to you. If you run a business, you have a duty to look after yourself, for your team, your clients, your family and business at the end of the day. Being a leader is about setting the precedents, showing what is expected through your actions. Showing them, they don't have to work all those hours. If you look after them, they will give back to you tenfold.

Another part of our culture that is incredibly damaging is this 'stiff upper lip' approach because it doesn't work.

Pretending something isn't happening isn't brave or stoic, it's denial. We can't ignore that burn-out is happening every day in our workplaces. We can't ignore that people are having breakdowns or that they are in burn-out. We are finally starting to break down the stigma of mental health. With 1 in 4 of us expected to struggle with mental health difficulties in our lifetime and the UN telling us that depression and anxiety will be the biggest global disease burden by 2030, we cannot afford to ignore it any longer.

While we're outing cultural expectations here, let's talk about those from our family and friends. How many of us feel guilty for taking time out for ourselves? We've got work to do, housework, shopping, washing and we want to be there for the kids before they go to bed. We're told consistently that we need to spend time with our partner or spouse because 'that's what you have to do' for a good relationship. Another good one is the promise of being able to "have it all" but sometimes you have to ask "at what cost?"

The 5am, hustle culture is rife within the high performers world and this sort of talk can often land people in a whole host of problems.

Nothing is worth sacficfing your health for, be it your mental, emotional, or physical health.

Where **do you fit in** there? Everyone needs time to replenish their energy cup and you are no different. There are no prizes for burning yourself out by doing everything everyone else needs.

Are you feeling bad going out with your friends when your hubby is at home?

Feeling guilty because you haven't seen your parents lately?

Grumpy because you ran out of time to bake cakes for your kid's class event and need to resort to supermarket offerings?

All of these things stop you from actually looking after yourself. How do you get rid of the guilt? When you give too much to everyone and don't fill up your cup, you end up feeling:

- *resentful*
- *bitter*
- *like you hate the situation or even the person*
- *like you're a victim*

We are going to use some tough love here. We're going to tell you what you **need** to hear, not what you want to hear. This might be uncomfortable but we're going to hold a mirror up so you can see the reality of what is happening.

The truth is that when you look after yourself and this can be as simple as

- *taking ten minutes for a cuppa*
- *reading for five minutes*
- *Having a workout*
- *meditating*
- *having a bath*
- *being with a pet, or*
- *putting a face mask on*

you become a better version of yourself. You transform from grumpy mum/dad to happy mum/dad, stressed Betty/Bob to positive Betty/Bob, resentful wife/husband to loving wife/husband. Just doing these simple things can literally transform your life and the lives of your family, friends and colleagues. So, you can see that it's your duty to do this for yourself to help those you care for and about.

Burn-out is still in its infancy in terms of how we deal with it. Not a lot of people recognise it or even acknowledge it. People who have come on our energy reset programme just see themselves as exhausted. Then we talk them through it on the programme and you can see it hit them in the face – this is me; this is what I feel like.

The great thing is that as soon as we recognise it and stop burying our heads in the sand, we can address it. We can turn it around and learn to manage our energy to be successful, happy, healthy, abundant and be optimistic and joyful again. That's how we all really want to feel.

6 PILLARS FOR A HAPPY AND HEALTHY LIFE

Critical to our energy reset programme are the 6 pillars we've identified. So many people fail in their efforts for a healthy and happy life because they don't base them on firm foundations. Each of our 6 pillars are critical to setting up those foundations to make your transformation achievable and sustainable. We want a transformation for you that stays for LIFE!

The first four relate to our ***physical health needs***:

Sleep

Sleep is the primary pillar for anything to do with health and energy management. It recharges our batteries, gets our brain clear and our body healed/recovered. No health or energy plan will succeed without prioritising sleep.

It's first because it's the most important factor for energy. If we haven't had enough quality sleep then we will not have enough energy throughout the day to make good cognitive decisions, or even to exercise.

A lot of people will go straight for nutrition or training for movement but if you haven't slept properly then none of that is going to happen. You're going to make bad decisions; your body is not going to want to move at all and you may even injure yourself.

Nobody who has a bad night's sleep wakes up feeling like a Disney princess/prince the next day. Working shift work has shown us just how much sleep can affect our cognition levels. Sleep deprivation can make you more emotionally vulnerable, bring down your emotional barriers and even make you a bit paranoid or react differently to things that wouldn't usually bother you. Our reserves are lower after a lack of sleep and therefore our capacity to deal with things is also reduced. There have been some studies showing that if you have a sleep debt of just 45 minutes it will decrease your cognitive function by 10-15%.

Water

Water and hydration are next. Our body is made up of 60 - 70% water depending on whether you are male or female. The earth is made up of 70% water and we understand the universe is believed to be 70% water. There's some sort of significant correlation in how energy is transferred through water.

Water is also the conduit that carries the nutrients around your body from your food. Dehydration can also cause headaches, and can reduce strength and cause brain fog. All things we don't want to experience.

Nutrition

Once you've addressed your sleep and you are hydrated then we talk about nutrition. If you're hearing 'diet' in your head right now, we want to tell you that you'll never hear us talk about diets. We concentrate on nourishing our bodies. When we concentrate on nourishing ourselves it makes us think about what we're putting into our body rather than just 'going on a diet'. When you think about eating kale instead of chocolate, that's about what food types you're eating. We focus on how we are nourishing our bodies and what it is doing for them.

Movement

Our body is like a machine and it's designed to move. Our philosophy is that it's not about exercising; it's about moving and being functional with our bodies. You're going to want to move your body. We always call it movement rather than exercise because it's movement that our bodies really need. Baz talks about two types of movement. The first one is physical activity – where we are active every day. We spend so much of our days being stagnant and sedentary at our desks. So, it's about walking up and down the stairs, parking a bit further from the supermarket, doing a bit of gardening and housework. The second, exercise, is where we move our body with a specific goal of being fitter and healthier.

Our body can reflect our emotions. If we've been sitting at a desk, stagnant, hunched over your computer – chances are you're feeling depressed and low. Our physiology affects our psychology and vice versa. Whereas if you get up and move about, start to exercise or have a bit of a walk then you will stand taller, hold your shoulders back and you're going to start feeling better about yourself.

Try it out now. go outside, stand up, look up. I challenge you not to feel happier. Put a smile on your face and try to feel depressed. You can't – it's impossible, isn't it? Now lower your shoulders and put a frown on your face. It's difficult to feel happy now, isn't it? The way we move our body can really affect our energy and how we approach our days.

The last two of our pillars relate to our ***mental wellbeing***:

Thought management

This pillar is about how we think and talk to ourselves. How do we talk to others? How do we see the world around us? What have we been told by others about ourselves that we have simply accepted as being true? What stories have we told ourselves? That we are lazy, not good enough, not clever enough? For some of us our parents or teachers have made comments that we have assumed to be correct and so many of us have carried those stories as truths, without stopping to question whether there is any evidence. Or we have made assumptions about ourselves that we have never stopped to reconsider their validity. Our thoughts are incredibly powerful.

DeStress/MeTime

Our last pillar is about filling our cup. This is a really big one when it comes to energy management. Most of us don't take time out to destress or engage in hobbies that make us feel good. In fact, we have trouble setting time aside to do the things we want to do, because we feel guilty or we struggle to relax. Maybe we think that writing, painting, colouring-in, swimming,playing tennis or surfing will take too much time. But there are things we can do that will only take five or ten minutes throughout the day just to take a breath, or to hit pause on our work and other responsibilities. So often we become the business owner or career person and we forget we are separate from our jobs, we forget who we are outside of our professional role. That DeStress/MeTime enables us to get back in contact with who we really are and provides the balance we really need in our lives.

Which brings us to what we're going to cover in the next five chapters.

OVERVIEW OF THE ENERGY RESET PROGRAMME

We've taken these 6 pillars and developed a comprehensive ***Five step Energy Reset programme***. These steps are incredibly important to make sustainable changes to the way you manage your energy.

Step 1 - The Space - Accept and Acknowledge
Step 2 - The Insight - Create Massive Awareness
Step 3 - The Permission - Taking INTENTIONAL Action
Step 4 - The Focus - Assessing and Adjusting
Step 5 - The Connection - Accelerating your results

So many people who are looking to change their energy levels or take any action to make a change, move straight to step three which is ***ACTION***. They try to move forward without really identifying the problem or taking stock of where they are at. Because they lack time, they just want to 'fix it", but that way you are just adding other actions to an already busy and stressful life when you are exhausted.

Steps one and two are so critical to building a path of sustainable change and we have seen the transformation in our clients. With any lasting change we need to take time to sit back and ask ourselves what is really going on. If you have a big decision to make with your business, career or life, you don't just take action without accessing all of the information you need, so you can make the best possible decision, before moving forward in the right way. Taking the time and space to ***accept and acknowledge*** what is really happening in your life is critical. If you're going to fix a problem then it's a no-brainer that you need to understand the exact problem you're trying to fix. The insight is where we do an assessment and an audit of where we are currently spending our energy. It's where we discover whether we are carrying an energy overdraft, meaning we are starting every day on the back foot in energy terms. These two steps give us the knowledge and understanding to move forward to step three which is about taking action.

Think about an archer, sniper or golfer. They don't just shoot and hope they hit their target. They consider their environment, the wind speed, temperature and the distance between them and their target. They will very likely fail if they simply aim and fire.

If you're trying to decide whether to take the time for these steps and you're tempted just to jump forward to step three, remember this quote from Henry Ford. *'If you always do what you've always done, then you'll always get what you've always got.'* If you want to feel different then take these tried and tested steps with us and you'll be feeling amazing in no time.

So, how did we come up with these five steps? They've come from the care plan that we followed for Loz's mental health. We've used them as a blueprint for absolutely every decision we make to move forward in our life.

When Loz had her breakdown in 2017 it was very much a case of just saying, right, what is actually going on here. We had no choice but to create the space and step back and look at what we'd been doing, with no judgement against ourselves for the choices we'd made. Then we asked ourselves more questions to be fully aware of everything influencing what was happening. That comes from our police and prison background where you'd turn up to a crime scene and assess the situation, considering all of the variables. We'd talk to witnesses and check CCTV, getting all of the evidence together before we made a call on how to proceed. We became the detectives in our own lives.

Based on all of the evidence, we then looked at permission. We had to give ourselves permission to take intentional action and determine where there might be subconscious objections to change. Then we'd take each piece, for example Loz's depression and ask ourselves why is it happening? What's going on? Then we'd decide what action we needed to take to address the depression. We'd try our approach for a few days and then evaluate if and how it was working. Then we'd focus in, adjust and assess the strategy. Is it working or not? If we're not making progress then we'd get help from the doctor or crisis team which is the next step – the next connection – about who you have around you in your life, and who your support structure is. To succeed in any area of our lives we need people around us who are on the same or similar journeys to us and we look a lot at that in step five.

Here is the outline of the 5 steps to powerfully aligning your energy:

Step One: The Space – Accept and Acknowledge

This chapter is all about accepting and acknowledging where you are at without judgement. The whole of the programme is about giving you this space. We all like to think we look at these things. We tell ourselves we really want to work on our health and that we really want to work on our energy, but we never actually give ourselves that space and time.

The only times we tend to do that is when we take part in training; when we're being coached; or when we're working with an accountability partner. We want you to give yourselves this space and honour yourselves enough to be able to really throw yourselves into this.

If we don't give it to ourselves then burnout is likely to happen. It's when you haven't looked after yourself and your body tells you you're going to take space or you'll pop. This is what happened with Loz. She went bang because she didn't acknowledge and accept what was going on. Her body and her mind stopped her until she took the space and time. We'd rather you take it on your own terms than letting your body do it for you by simply stopping.

Step Two: The Insight – Create Massive Awareness

This is where we look at awareness and at how you're going to manage your actual energy. It's going to be really interesting for you when we start to look at what some of the signs and symptoms that are turning up for you are. This step is the process that is often missed out but it holds vital clues to what is really going on. It can sometimes be an ugly step, as you might find out some things you don't want to hear. However, we can promise you that this step will enlighten you and empower you to feel good about finally having all the information you need to then take a huge leap into the next step.

Step Three: The Permission – Taking Intentional Action
This chapter is going to be a big one for a lot of you. It's about the permission. This is all about taking action, without guilt. You may even feel guilty for taking the time to read and action what's in this book. We'll help by talking about overcoming objections so you can get moving.

The other thing we will talk to you about in this step is ***intentional action***. When we take action from a place of intention the results are much more powerful. This step will blow your socks off!

Step Four: The Focus – Assess and Adjust
In this chapter we're going to assess and adjust your strategy to make sure it's actually working. We all have strategies for our businesses and careers to keep them healthy and we factor in time to assess and adjust these. But do you do it for yourself and your health and wellbeing?

I am sure in the past you have started something and then stopped, because "something happened". Right or wrong? This stage of assessing and adjusting using focus will ensure that you never stop because 'something happened', and that you use strategies to keep you moving forward. At the end of the day that's what you want, right?

Step Five: The Connection – Accelerate your result
Here we'll look at how you can accelerate your results and in life. You can do this in relation to the people around you and the information you're taking in. They say that we are the sum of the

5 people we hang about with. We believe this to be true both physically and virtually.

If you want to accelerate your results and keep this going, this step - The Connection will be crucial for you.

Before you start on chapter three, we want you to take a minute to remember the pact you made with yourself earlier in this book.

You are going to find recognising some of this uncomfortable. But there is no room for judgement in this process, all that will do is stop you being honest with yourself. Just accept and acknowledge what is happening – that is the critical first step to fixing it. The chances are that you were trying hard to do all you could for your career, business and family. We will help you through our energy reset programme to manage your energy better so that you can be the best you that you can be.

You got this! Let's get started.

CHAPTER THREE

The Space

For us to know where
we are going we must
first know where we truly
are, wholeheartedly,
and without judgement

Laura and Barry Ash

Now we've covered what burn-out is and we know about the 3 dimensions – let's start to create some space where we can accept and acknowledge where we're at right now.

This is about taking a step back to take a huge, powerful step forwards into empowerment.

You may not realise it but even just knowing this has given you some power back. This knowledge can put you in control right now because you get it, you see it - it's there right in front of you.

So, if you feel a bit rubbish about the boxes you ticked when we looked at the 3 dimensions of burn-out give yourself a pat on the back because it takes a lot of guts to admit to these.

So often we see these problems in our minds but we think that the answer is to just keep pushing. But the more we push against something the more resistance we'll get back. We talk a lot about energy in this – if we push our energy barriers then we're definitely going to get something back. We've got to take a step back and release that pressure, so we can see the bigger picture. Once we see the bigger picture and we're not under the same pressure we can deal more effectively with the situations that arise.

Acknowledge and accept without judgement

The reason we've got step one in place is **to accept and acknowledge and take a step back** is because whenever we've worked with people with mental health problems, or alcohol or drug addictions, the very first step is to accept and to acknowledge where you are right now.

But one of the most important things to do here is to

Be open and honest and not judge yourself.

There's no need to complain or explain. Be brave enough to admit it. We can so often feel like we're imposters, that we are let downs, weak or useless. It's usual for these beliefs to show themselves. But it takes a stronger, braver, more warrior-like person to recognise these feelings than to hide away from them.

We really want to encourage and empower you to say yes - this is what is going on with me. When you complain or try to explain, you avoid taking responsibility for what's happening in your life. It's you trying to pass the buck. As soon as we open up and accept it, we take responsibility for it and then we can take action.

Energy can only contain one space. We talk about this a lot when we talk about moving things forward. If you're not prepared to get rid of this old, stagnant, burned-out energy and you're not prepared to accept it and acknowledge it, then it will always be there waiting to be dealt with before you can actually move forwards.

We need to get it, lift it, ditch it and put another sort of energy in that space – a new more abundant energy, one that is going to make you more powerful, that will propel you forward, not only to make you happier and healthier, but to bring more abundance into your career and more money into your business.

Let us ask you this. How can you possibly have new things come into your life if you are still holding on to the old things? You need to make some room for the new, good and exciting energy to flow!

Whatever you want to create, you can't create it from an energy that is about loss, less and lack. Nine times out of ten we come at this from a place of fear and a sense of lack. It's normal in that space to cling desperately to things. But the problem is that we've got to think about what it is we're putting out into the world and what are we creating from and getting back from this energy? What you're going to create from that energy is more of the sense of lack and therefore more fear. So, we need to be able to accept and acknowledge and see it for what it is.

Ask yourself – what is it at this very moment that I want to create?

What is the energy I want to have present right now in my life to move forward?

We can think of energy like water in a bottle. If we keep the water in the bottle (or the energy in our bodies) and it doesn't flow then what happens to the water in the bottle? It becomes stagnant. When energy doesn't flow freely it also becomes stagnant. Stagnant water is no good for anybody and the same is true of stagnant energy. So, we have to allow energy in and to flow through and out of us. We can't let energy sit still in our bodies. A lot of us think we're lacking energy so we're going to do nothing. But by doing nothing we become stagnant. We need to do something. We don't need to run a marathon but we have to do something to get rid of the negative energy so it allows space for new energy to flow in.

'If we don't acknowledge it's there – how can we hope to change it?'

ENERGY EXERCISE

Picture your body. What energy do you want to be made up of?

Look at this first empty water bottle.

Think about the energy you have and are feeling right now. Use your words or colours to fill it in

Be as creative as you want but be honest with yourself.

You might want to use red for anger, or black for sluggishness.

You might want to draw a cloud to represent a foggy head or draw squiggles to represent how busy your mind feels.

You might decide to use words and write how you feel in the bottle.

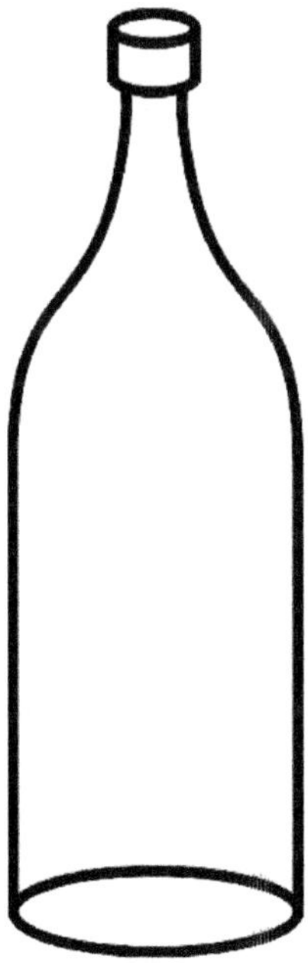

Now take a look at this second water bottle. It's so full of potential.

This one represents what you WANT to feel like. What energy do you want your body to be filled with?

Just like the first one, use words and colours to fill it up.

Be as creative as you like and just go with it.

You might want to draw a sun for energy or draw a smiley face.

You may want to use energetic colours of green, purple, or pink. You might even want to draw the Chakras if you're into that sort of thing.

Use empowering words to describe how you WANT to feel.

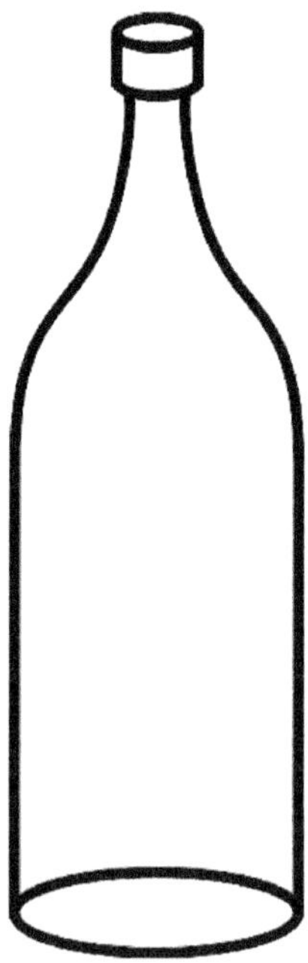

Just take a step back and look at the two bottles for a minute and compare them.

> **This bottle only has space for so much energy. If you want it to be like bottle 2 then you need to get rid of the energy in bottle 1.**

What are some of the things that stop us from creating the space we want?

- *Fear*
- *Having to actually do something about it*
- *It becomes real*
- *Weakness*
- *Judgement from ourselves and others*

Most of us understand and recognise fear but it's a huge step to realise we need to actually do something about it. When we own up to ourselves and admit that this is what's going on, we are compelled to act and that's quite scary sometimes. For most of us we are our own worst critic, so it's the judgement from ourselves that is hardest to face.

Face Everything And Rise

We know that you will rise up and step into the powerhouse that you really are. You're a diamond underneath it all. You just need a little shaking off, dusting down and buffing on the edges to bring out your sparkle and you will be brighter than ever.

ACTIVITY

So, this is what we want you to do now, if you haven't already.

1. **From a non-judgemental space we want you to look at the 3 dimensions of burn-out. Which ones can you most identify with now and in the past?**

You can tick them off in the table below.

PHYSICAL/EXHAUSTION

Feelings of being worn out	
Loss of energy	
Feeling depleted	
Total fatigue	
Lack of motivation	
Limited physical movement	

CYNICISM/MENTAL

Being negative or having an inappropriate attitude towards others	
Irritable	
Loss or belief in others and the world	
Withdraw from society	

POWERLESSNESS/EMOTIONAL

Feelings of reduced personal achievement	
Reduced productivity	
Reduced feelings of capability	
Low morale	
Inability to cope with every day	

After you've done that and acknowledged that that is what is going on for you then tell yourself this, out loud or write it down if you want to that

> I [insert your name here] am now making the commitment, the intention, and the decision to move all this aside without judgement because it no longer serves me. I [insert your name here] am ready to create something new.

Next up it's time to replace that energy. Remember we spoke about getting rid of the old to welcome in the new, this is where this happens for you now.

2. **After releasing that energy, we need to replace it with a powerful affirmation.**

Replace it with an affirmation that really resonates with you, one that you can feel deep in your gut.

Remember energy never sits still, it's always changing and transferring and moving about. So, let's replace it with something more powerful and self-affirming. Something that is going to bring more and more of the positive energy you want in your life towards you.

This is how you move on from that stagnant, negative, burn out energy to attracting more positive and abundant energy into your life. It's now time to move on and start looking forward.

Let's replace 'I feel tired', 'I feel stressed' with more powerful, positive energy because as soon as you start changing your language it will start to change your life because that will be the energy you put out into the world and it will come back to you in spades.

Some options might be:

'I am mutating the old into a positive new energy'

'I have the tools I need to move forward with abundance'.

'I am enough.'

'I am the creator of my own journey'

What is your affirmation? What will positively reinforce you on this energy reset journey?

We would suggest that you sit for a few moments, perhaps with your eyes closed and feel what it feels like to BE this affirmation. How it feels, perhaps what colour it is, where you feel the energy in your body and imagine it getting brighter and brighter for you. Imagine it gets so bright that it blows away the stagnant energy BAM!

Put this affirmation where you will see it the most and read it several times a day while closing your eyes and affirming this feeling to yourself

We have something a little extra for you to do tonight AND for the rest of the steps if you are up for the challenge.

The challenge!

We challenge you to not look at your phone 1 hour before you go to bed and for 1 hour after you wake up in the morning.

Leave it alone, give yourself some time to yourself and see how it feels.

Remember the world won't implode if you take some time awa

WHAT'S NEXT?

In chapter four we'll be looking at The Insight; Energy versus Money; Awareness with the 3 dimensions of burnout in relation to our 6 pillars of health and wellbeing.

CHAPTER FOUR

The Insight

The quality of your life is a direct reflection of the quality of the questions you are asking yourself

---

Tony Robbins

Let's recap before we dive right into step 2 for you.

In step one we talked about ***the space*** and taking the time to accept and acknowledge where we are right now, without judgement. We hope by now you can understand why it's such an important place to start because if we don't even give ourselves the space to acknowledge our reality, then it's unlikely we'll prioritise time and space to fix the problem.

You've had 24 hours to let it sink in. How did you find it? How did your extra challenge go to avoid your phone for an hour before bed and after you got up in the morning?

Most people find the phone challenge, well, a challenge! However once they do it, they find that it just free's up a bit of real estate in their minds. They find they sleep better, pick up a book or even just have a bath. It's important that we create a bit of breathing space for ourselves.

You can record your results here if you like. You can use it to compare to how you're doing by the end of these steps.

This chapter is all about insight. We're going to delve deeper into awareness and we'll be asking you whether you are an energy saver, an energy spender or an energy investor?

We're going to put a typical day under a microscope and see where you are spending and gaining your energy. It's a tool we use for ourselves and our clients and it's a real eye opener.

Then we'll take you through the 3 dimensions of burn-out alongside our 6 pillars with deeper insight in mind.

This is a crucial step, because as you know most people will jump right to ACTION with a diet, new workout regime or some fad diet which we all know is going to land you back at square one. This step is going to help you ask questions to get a deeper understanding as to where you are and what actually needs working on.

We want you to put your Detective Specs on and really look at what is going on around you. When Loz was in the Police Force and had to attend a scene, she had to collate all the evidence to hand over the case for it to be investigated. She would collect witness statements, CCTV and SOCO (scene of crime officers) would attend. Then when she moved to an investigative role the aim was a prosecution so that involved so much more digging and evidence gathering.

However, this evidence gathering made it easy for our team to determine the next steps in the case.

If you have ever had to make an important decision in your life, what have you done? Weighed up the pros and cons, did some research, and asked a bunch of questions. Why? because you wanted all the information EVEN if it was obvious.

This is exactly the same. Your health is a very important part of your life and as such should be treated like this.

Imagine an archer with a bow and arrow. Perhaps Robin Hood, or Katniss Everdeen. Before they take their shot, they pull BACK the arrow, look at wind direction, lighting and distance before they take the shot. Then POW with all this information AND the pulling back of the arrow they take their shot and BAM they hit a bullseye.

That's enough of that, let's get started!

ENERGY VERSUS MONEY

Theophrastus, who was a pal of Aristotle's, said that

'Time is the most valuable thing a man can spend'.

Given they lived more than two thousand years ago, it is a fact that is just as relevant, if not more, than it was back then.

It's a no-brainer then that we completely agree with this idea. Time is very much like money. If you don't allocate money, it will just get spent. Time is exactly the same. So many of us are waiting until the end of the month for our money or income to be replenished.

You need to allocate every penny and its place otherwise it will just disappear. It's the same with time and energy. If we're not allocating or spending it, it will just get wasted. That doesn't mean we have to be really reserved about our time and the way we spend it. But it's very valuable to have a clear view on how and where you're spending your time and how that's affecting your energy.

If we gave you £1000 today, what would you do with it? (Disclaimer – we are NOT giving all of our readers £1000. Sorry about that.)

Would you...

- *Save it?*
- *Spend it all at once?*
- *Give it away?*
- *Spend it slowly?*
- *Invest it?*

Would you spend it slowly and be really frugal with it? Or would you be frivolous and spend it all in one go. Or you could invest it.

Have a think about what your first instinct would be. Which would you do?

You can write it down here.

____

____

____

____

Some of you might think that you'll save it and then spend it all at once. Or you might think you'll get that handbag you've been hankering for and get some flowers for somebody. You might decide to invest it. You might choose 2 or 3 of these options. You might save, spend and give some away for example.

The reason you are likely to be able to answer this question quite quickly is because you understand the value of money. We always use this analogy when we work with business owners and corporations because generally people understand the value of money, so it's something we can all relate to. If you can understand the value of money and allocation and spending it then you can use this to understand the value of time and energy.

Sometimes we know what to do, but do we always act on that knowledge? Are you matching your knowledge with action? No-one always does the sensible thing but knowing and acting on that knowledge are completely different things and both are essential.

We're going to have a look at a typical day equating money to energy. We've done some simple maths on this so you can consider what the typical day of someone experiencing burn-out looks like.

Starting point £1000

		£1000
Wake up, check emails	-£50	£950
No time for breakfast	-£100	£850
Rush to work, a lot to do	-£50	£800
Work all morning, no time for breaks	-£100	£700
Work through lunch, trying to catch up, don't eat and no break	-£200	£500
Work all afternoon with no break	-£100	£400
You leave for home and you're knackered	-£100	£300
Don't feel like cooking so have something 'quick', make a crappy meal or order takeaway & eat crappy meal	-£150	£150
Have some downtime with friends/family	+£100	£250
Go to bed late, exhausted with only one crappy meal all day	-£100	£150
Too much on your mind, can't wind down so you have a sleepless night	-£750	-£600
	Daily total	-£600
	Work week total	-£3000

Let's break this example day down a little more.

How many of us are checking our work emails as soon as we wake up? That gets us focused immediately on work and because of that we already feel behind so we rush headlong into work without a good breakfast and a chance to wake up properly. All of that is coming out of our 'energy bank'.

If we've already decided that we're behind in our work we compound the problem by skipping breaks and lunch. We may not even realise as we leave work exhausted, that we haven't eaten all day. Or we've used caffeine or chocolate to 'get us through' those last few hours.

At home, assuming we've even had the time or energy to get the shopping in, we've all eaten cheese on toast and pretended it's a meal. We might get some great energy back from spending time with our family/friends. For some of us though, that might take energy we don't have as well. If we're feeling guilty about not having a proper meal or we've missed bath time or bedtime, that guilt is going to spend more of the depleted energy in our 'account'.

Exhaustion, guilt and anxiety are not great bedfellows and for many of us sleep can be elusive. Our mind rushes through all the things we need to do or haven't done from the day, making slumber impossible. Our body needs that time to regenerate and recuperate. If we don't get it then we start the next day exhausted. Ironically the more we push ourselves, the more exhausted we get, the less productive we are.

LET'S TALK ABOUT YOUR TYPICAL DAY...

Does this sample day remind you of how yours feel? Does it look vaguely familiar? Does it feel like we've been following you around with a camera? Be honest with yourself. Remember there is no room for judgement here. We're just looking at how it is, not making any judgement on whether it's good or bad.

How often does this happen? How many of your work days feel like this? If it looks like your average working day then how does that make you feel?

So, let's consider this exercise again. At the beginning of the day, we gave you £1000 in energy to spend. You've spent a total of £1600, so your balance is at -£600. You are overdrawn by £600.

More than that – not getting a good night's sleep means you start the day with a minus of £600 in your energy balance. Can you imagine what the next day is going to be like?

If you carry on living the same day for one week, you are going to be overdrawn by £3000 in your energy bank balance by the end of the working week. In fact, it's probably going to look worse than that because starting each day with a deficit in your bank balance is going to mean you are having to work twice as hard to focus and produce anything in your workplace. And if you work more than five days a week it will be higher again.

You can see by looking at just one week how burn-out can hit us so quickly. We are spending more than we are earning. Nobody likes to be in the red at the end of the day. Would you accept your bank balance being overdrawn to that extent every day? It's unlikely.

However, in this crazy world we live in so very many of us live our lives 'in the red' in our energy accounts.

CAN YOU AFFORD TO BE CARRYING THIS EVER-GROWING ENERGY 'DEBT'?

What are the consequences of being 'in the red'?

- *Tired*
- *Snappy*
- *Get sick more easily and often*
- *Unable to concentrate*
- *Foggy mind*
- *Flitting*
- *Never finish a job*
- *Poor work quality*
- *Frustration*
- *Anxiety*
- *Depression*
- *BANG BURN-OUT HITS*

You can see how that mounts up so easily. If we equate that energy to money, we can see how our energy is being spent throughout the day.

It's so helpful to see our energy in terms of money because we can picture it and understand it in a practical way. We can imagine having that money in our hands to spend. We can see it when we spend it and earn it in a really tangible way. We're guessing that looking at it like this this has been a bit of a shock to you.

This is a real education in managing your energy - right here!

Energy is a little bit different because we let it go without having the same physical reminder as we do it. But putting it in terms of money we can understand how quickly we are spending it. It makes us realise where we are spending our energy.

Whenever we spend money, we always know we're going to replenish it. If you're a business owner you'll do a campaign or promotion to bring more business in. If you work for someone you know that your wage or salary will be coming in to cover your expenditure.

The problem with energy is how to replenish it. How can you fill your cup with energy again as you spend it? Happily, this is what this book is about.

Let's have a look at someone who might spend their energy a bit more consciously.

		£1000
Wake up and have breakfast, have time to get yourself 'into the day'	+£50	£1050
Go to work, no need to rush. Cool, calm & confident.	+£50	£1100
You work all morning	-£100	£1000
Have a short break – take time to move around or clear your head	+£50	£1050
Take a lunch break – nourish yourself, close your laptop & go to a different environment	+£200	£1250
Work in the afternoon, clear headed and refuelled	-£100	£1150
Have an afternoon break, even 5 or 10 minutes	+£50	£1200
Get home from work and cook a meal	-£50	£1150
Eat your meal – relax, take time to digest	+£50	£1200
Time out with your family chilling out	+£100	£1300
Calm bedtime routine – go to bed in time to get enough rest. Disconnect from day and devices.	+£250	£1550
	Daily total	+£1550
	Work week total	+£7750

It's a no-brainer that going into your day with a credit from the day before is much more attractive.

Let's just have a look at the findings about fatigue alone in the workplace, from this piece of research:

> *'It has influences directly on many people's physical and mental abilities needed to carry out even simple tasks. The most important effects of fatigue include decreased task motivation, longer reaction time, reduction of alertness, impaired concentration, poorer psychometric coordination, problems in memory and information processing, and poor judgement. It is estimated that fatigue in workplaces is costing more than 18 billion $ a year in the US.'*[3]

Not looking after yourself is costing your business and your organisation money and it's affecting the quality of your work.

Let's have a look at your typical day. Use this chart to list what you usually do on your working days. Be honest, it will give you a really good indication of where you are spending your energy and where you are getting it back.

What we usually do:

What would your ideal day look like?

Can you see how different just a few small breaks and nourishment can make to your energy account?

Can we just interject here and just say stop thinking about HOW this will happen? You're probably thinking "I'll never be able to change this," "I don't have the time," "what are they talking about!" Let us assure you that this can be done, we have methods that are simple. This step is all about just asking questions and NOT taking action.

We know that you probably want to jump straight to that because

1. **It's what you have always done**
2. **You're a highly driven person.**

We just want to put the reins on you and slow you down here from those racing thoughts – okay?

The consequences of managing your energy and your day are going to be:

- *Better clarity*
- *More energy*
- *More productive*
- *No flitting*
- *At peace*
- *Happier*
- *Healthier*
- *No BANG!*
- *Skipping down the road!*

So, you can see the huge difference in the way you function during the day. Taking time out for some headspace, calm, a change of environment and to nourish yourself physically and emotionally will have you in energy credit.

Did you notice that in example two you would be in credit to the tune of £7750 instead of in debit £3000 in your energy account?

There's a good chance earlier in this chapter when we talked about spending money that you decided you might spend some of the £1000 in cash we talked about. If you were more conscious about adding energy into your day it's very likely you would be much more confident about spending your energy when you needed or wanted to, if you finished most days in credit.

THIS MOVES US NICELY ON TO STEP 2.

Now that we can see in practical terms what energy management looks like, we're going to move onto the insight. This is about **creating massive awareness** and auditing your lifestyle, time spent and the people around you. This will help reveal the truth about what is going on in your life.

A big part of why we want to start with acceptance and acknowledgement, and then move on to awareness, is because the ultimate objective is to really help you manage your energy.

When we were managing Loz's health after her 2017 big bang, we realised just how much was about how we dealt with her bipolar. When we looked at addressing her mental health it was all about energy management.

The first part was acknowledging where she was really at and accepting it without judging herself for choices she'd made or things she hadn't done.

The second part is so much about awareness. It's about putting on the detective specs and really looking at what is going on in our life. We need to detect our triggers and symptoms because we both believe that if we don't know what's really going on and haven't looked at it, we can't move forward because we're trying to move forward on rocky ground and with dodgy foundations. As we said earlier, in the police service we would create massive awareness by investigating the case – we'd collect all of the evidence and then once we had all of that, we could then move on and then make a case or informed decision about what we needed to. Otherwise, we're just bouncing around from pillar to post and guessing what we should be doing.

Having *awareness* is such a huge part of creating change. It's so important to do our self-audit.

What does your day look like? Where are you using your energy? Where are you creating your energy? When you know this, you can start manifesting the energy you want and need to propel you forward to be what you really want to be.

We need **situational awareness**. In our coaching programmes we always spend time on this. We ask in depth questions to work out what's really happening in your life and where you are spending and investing in your energy on a daily basis. It's great to be able to do it that way.

So, your job now, reading this book, is to put your detective specs on.

If you're thinking that doing nothing might be an option, sadly that's not true. Staying still doesn't work because the energy in your body will get stagnant and stale. Your body can't add fresher, more positive energy if it's already full of stale and stagnant energy.

Remember that it's vital to understand that you need to take things steadily and sustainably. It's so important in this process to identify triggers and symptoms in relation to your energy. They could be holding you back but once you know what they are then you can sort them out.

LET'S HAVE A LOOK AT THE INSIGHT AND CREATING MASSIVE AWARENESS IN LINE WITH THE 6 PILLARS.

Pull out your journal or flip back in the book and check which dimension of burn-out you aligned with the most yesterday:

- *Physical/Exhaustion*
- *Mental/Cynicism*
- *Emotional/Powerlessness*

This will really help you to get the most out of the next exercise.

PHYSICAL/EXHAUSTION

In chapter one we talked about exhaustion. This is the physical phase where you feel depleted and empty. So, the way we would tackle exhaustion would be with the first 4 pillars (P) of health and wellbeing which are **sleep, water, food and exercise**.

This is how we deal with the exhaustion dimension of burn-out. These are the things you need to be asking yourself to understand what is happening for you and to create awareness.

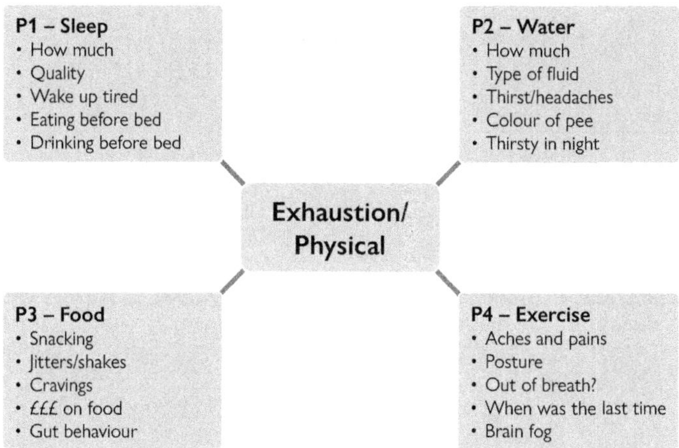

PILLAR 1- SLEEP

Some of the things you need to consider in relation to your sleep are:

- ☐ *How much sleep are you getting?*
- ☐ *What quality of sleep are you having?*
- ☐ *Are you waking up tired?*
- ☐ *Are you eating before bed because if we eat just before we sleep, especially high levels of sugar or alcohol, our body has to process that?*

Our body only has a certain amount of energy to work at night. Because at night its role is rest and recuperation. If it's digesting food then that's taking away valuable energy our body needs for recuperation. Digesting food takes up a massive amount of energy, but we need it to draw from. So eating earlier in the evening means that your body can rest while it's sleeping.

These are some of the signs and symptoms you can use to ask yourself, is this happening to me? Am I ticking off some of these? Investigate this and be curious.

You can record your answers here.

____

____

____

____

____

____

PILLAR 2 - WATER/HYDRATION

These are the key things to think about in terms of hydration and water:

- ☐ *How much fluid are you drinking during the day?*
- ☐ *What type of fluid are you drinking?*

- ☐ *Are you reaching for the energy or caffeinated drinks?*
- ☐ *Or are you going for the pure and simple H2O?*
- ☐ *Are you getting headaches from being thirsty?*
- ☐ *Look at the colour of your pee – does it look like a pint of Guinness, a glass of orange juice or does it look a pale straw colour?*
- ☐ *Where are you sitting on the scale?*
- ☐ *Are you getting thirsty at night?*
- ☐ *Are you waking up with a dry mouth?*

Remember what we talked about in the last chapter about the 3 dimensions of burn-out? If you identify with exhaustion, these are some of the things you need to be aware of, and to ask yourself questions about, to identify your symptoms.

An easy way to check your hydration levels is to check out the colour of your pee. If it's darker on the scale from straw coloured to Guinness then drinking some more water is a great idea. If you wake up tired then you might need to look at how much sleep you're getting.

You can see that these are really simple things to do that we often miss because we believe it has to be complicated, and it does not need to be.

Are any of these resonating with you? Feel free to record your answers here.

____

____

____

____

PILLAR 3 - FOOD

It's most helpful to look at these points about food and nourishment:

- [ ] *Ask yourself if you're snacking unnecessarily?*
- [ ] *Do you need to have something next to you while you're working?*
- [ ] *What's in your bin - biscuit wrappers?*
- [ ] *Are you getting the jitters or the shakes? What we mean by that is are you having sugar crashes where you start shaking a lot and feel like you need something sweet like a chocolate bar?*

We work with a lot of people who experience cravings. A lot of people in the corporate world feel as though in order to do a task they need to have a particular kind of food as a reward.

One big question is how much money are you spending on food? For example, when you're on the way home do you think 'I might just get a bottle of wine on the way'. Or might you decide to order takeaway that night? Have you audited your money and seen how much you're spending on takeaways and alcohol?

Let's get down to the serious business of gut behaviour. How many times do you poo every day or week? Do you get constipation or IBS (irritable bowel syndrome)? All of these things are going to affect your physical exhaustion and your ability to cope during the day. If you have a strong body and strong health foundations then burn-out is much less likely to happen. If you're ticking a lot of these boxes, your body is going to be energy depleted and you're going to have to create more energy to try and deal with some of these symptoms.

Note down any of these that are happening for you here.

____

____

____

____

____

____

PILLAR 4 - EXERCISE

Exercise and movement are critical to our energy – are any of these happening for you right now?

- ☐ *Is your body full of aches and pains constantly?*
- ☐ *Do you get a lot of back, ankle, knee or hip pain?*

- ☐ *What is your posture like? Our posture and our energy are so connected.*
- ☐ *Are you out of breath all the time?*
- ☐ *Are you in fight or flight?*
- ☐ *When was the last time you actually did something physical?*
- ☐ *Have you been putting physical activity off for a long time?*
- ☐ *Are you getting brain fog?*
- ☐ *Are you finding it hard to concentrate?*

Think about your body as a car engine. If you don't start your car up for a while the battery goes flat. A lot of people think they need energy to exercise, in actual fact exercise gives you energy. It's another great way to get the stagnant energy out of our body which makes room for the good stuff. It doesn't have to be hard and fast exercise. It's just about moving your body - simple!.

Are you having any of these symptoms or signs? Record them here.

____

____

____

CYNICISM/MENTAL

If you found that cynicism was one you were really relating to in chapter one, then here are a few things you can consider: assessing where you are at, and creating a bit of awareness about what might be happening for you. We've broken these down into four parts – physical, input, output and internal.

If you related most to this then the way we deal with this is through pillar 5 which is 'Thought Management'.

Pillar 5 – Thought management

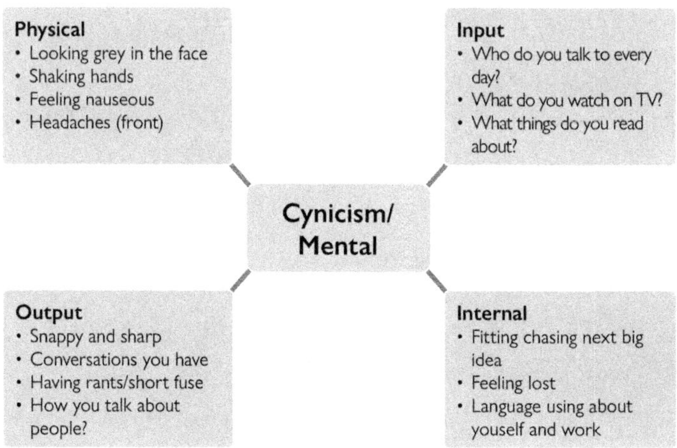

When we work with people or clients you will take them through a process like this to work out what's happening with them, and how you might best be able to help them. This process is similar.

So, you might notice:

PHYSICAL

- *Are you Looking grey in the face*
- *Do you have Shaking hands or having tremors*
- *Feeling nauseous or is your tummy upset*
- *Headaches in the front of your head, or tension headaches*

INPUT

- *Who do you talk to every day? How are people speaking to you? Are you picking up negative energy from other people?*
- *What do you watch on TV? Are you energised or drained from what you're watching on TV? Do dramas or soaps drain your energy?*
- *What things do you read about? It's great to know what's happening in the world, but are you reading or taking in too much bad news at once? Is this impacting you or making you feel tired?*

Be mindful of what you're absorbing and taking in. Watching the news can make you see and feel that the world can be a very negative place. That will affect your mental health and this cynicism part. Sometimes just by changing that and changing the input can change you, and lift you up and alter your energy in a positive way. These are small things that can really impact how we feel.

OUTPUT

- *Are you snappy and sharp (we call this Crocodile chat)?*
- *What conversations are you having?*
- *Are you having rants or have a short fuse?*
- *How are you talking about people?*

Just have a think and ask yourself these questions

- ☐ *How are you interacting with others?*
- ☐ *What energy are you putting out to the world?*
- ☐ *Are you feeling negative about people and seeing them in a negative way?*
- ☐ *Is this impacting on how you're communicating with them?*
- ☐ *Do you find you have a short fuse or ranting when you're speaking with others?*
- ☐ *What about when you are talking about other people?*
- ☐ *Are you feeling positive about them or are you feeling petty or judgemental?*

INTERNAL

- *Are you flitting or chasing the next big thing – are you prone to fad diets, or the latest advertised marketing plan?*
- *Are you feeling lost and losing sight of your purpose?*
- *What is the language you're using about yourself and work?*

Again, just have a think and ask yourself these questions

- [ ] *What language are you using about the way you're working and living?*
- [ ] *Are you feeling focussed and sure of your approach and vision?*
- [ ] *When you talk about your work or business are you conscious of using positive or negative words?*
- [ ] *When you're feeling unsure are you finding yourself wanting to try something new, to rush into the next 'big' thing?*

This is the pillar we refer to as thought management. The way we look at it is that the first 4 pillars are about your physical being and pillars 5 and 6 are about your mental wellbeing.

Is this happening for you?

____

____

____

____

____

____

POWERLESSNESS/EMOTIONAL

The last one is about our emotions. We might have imposter syndrome, we might be questioning our abilities and feeling really down on ourselves and our place in the world.

If you related most to this then the way we deal with this is through pillar 6 which is 'DeStress Me Time'.

Pillar 6 – DeStressMeTime

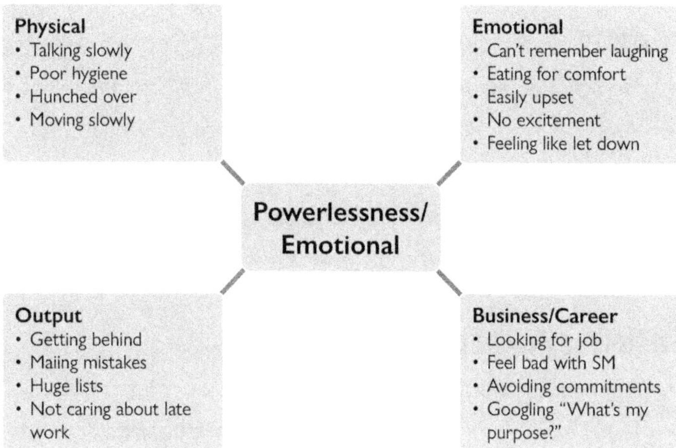

Like Mental/Cynicism we have divided this into 4 sections to really get a better look at what is going on

PHYSICAL

- *Are you talking slowly?*
- *Do you have poor hygiene?*
- *Are you hunched over?*
- *Are you moving slowly? Are you hiding yourself, or not feeling good?*

EMOTIONAL

- *Are you struggling to remember the last time you had a belly laugh?*
- *Are you eating for comfort?*
- *Are you getting upset easily?*
- *Is there nothing you're feeling excited about?*
- *Are you feeling like you've been let down?*

OUTPUT

- *Do you feel like you're getting behind in what you need to do?*
- *Are you making mistakes/doubting what you've done?*
- *Are your to-do lists becoming huge?*
- *Have you stopped caring about late work because you think it's going to be crap anyway?*

BUSINESS/CAREER

- *Are you looking for a job?*
- *Does looking at social media make you feel bad?*
- *Are you avoiding commitments?*
- *Are you Googling 'what's my purpose?' or 'is it normal to feel like this?'*

The energy feel of all of these is low. As we mentioned, don't look at these and rush ahead thinking about how you can fix this or make this work. We want you just to sit within this space and take the opportunity to look at the different areas of the 3 dimensions and ask the questions around the pillars. Which one do I really need to work on first?

It might take a little while, even a couple of days, to sit with this and contemplate the points. We know from our own experience that you need to let it percolate a little bit. Take your time with this bit – it is worth giving it enough time. If you do this properly and have all of the information you need then you can make a proper informed decision. In your business or career, you wouldn't normally make snap decisions on important topics. You would want to get all of the information and to know where you stand, this is no different. There is no bigger or more important subject than your health. You are the cog pivotal to all parts of you and you must give yourself time to work on this to get it right.

Record what you're experiencing in terms of powerlessness here.

____

____

____

____

____

So, by this stage you will know how to audit the 3 dimensions of burn-out in line with the 6 pillars from a non-judgemental or emotional space. You have completed the insight into what is happy in your life.

Remember not to try and fix it or take action YET!

Just consider ticking off or noting those things that resonate with you. It will give you an insight into the things that you most need to change.

If you try to take action on something you're unsure about you're not going to take the right action to solve the problems and that's going to be energy you don't have right now.

There is no action when we take an audit in our professional or personal lives. It's just to gain awareness of what is happening. It's about gathering as much information as we possibly can.

You can use a table like this and note down your findings

Exhaustion - Physical	**Cynical - Mental**	**Powerlessness - Emotional**
Sleep	Physical	Physical
Water	Input	Emotional
Food	Output	Output
Exercise	Internal	Business/Career

You might look at some of these and think that you're fine with some of them. You might look through cynicism and think I'm fine with all of these. Powerlessness, you might go through and think that there are some of the emotional factors that you resonate with. Physical, you may or may not be feeling right now. You'll get more in certain boxes than you will in others. That's why an audit is so important because one size does not fit all. You need to know what is happening in your life right now. It's just about recognising it and laying it out. We get that it can be a bit overwhelming to start with, but once you get into it, you'll find it feels less huge. We recommend you spend about 15-20 minutes looking at each one and thinking about it. Go back over the slides/tables/diagrams and ask yourself some of the questions. Put those detective specs on and have a look.

The next chapter is about permission. We talk about why it's so important to give yourself permission to take action. We look at any objections and resistance to moving forward. Then we'll look at some ideas for taking action on the 6 pillars and how you can create habits to make sustainable and positive changes in your life.

CHAPTER FIVE

The Permission

The only impossible journey is the one you never begin

Tony Robbins

This section is going to be huge. This is the stage where you'll feel that you want to leap in but you'll feel a bit guilty about it.

The Permission is all about being able to take guilt-free action and we're going to cover a lot of ground, including:

- *Objections to taking action*
- *Why giving yourself permission is so important*
- *The reality of taking action*
- *Our ethos for taking action*
- *Taking action in line with the 6 pillars and 3 dimensions*
- *Creating habits*

Before you move on to the permission, it's critical to have addressed Steps 1 and 2 . If you haven't already acted on The Space and The Insight then go back and do that now, before you move on. We all need to walk before we can run, and energy management is no different. To get the most out of all of this you must take each step in its place.

It's at this point if you have done Step 1 and 2 that it will really start to come into its own for you and prove useful. Usually, as you know, this would have been the step you jump to immediately and this is also the step that you STAY at all the time.

It's a great idea when you get to this point to sit back for a minute and work out how this is all sitting for you right now.

How are you feeling about what you've read in steps 1 and 2? What has particularly resonated for you?

OBJECTIONS TO TAKING ACTION

We've all been there. We've identified the problem we want to fix, we're ready to move forward but...well...nothing. We don't take action. Why is that? In the work we do with our clients and corporations we've heard so many of the reasons people don't take action on their health and wellbeing. These are some of the most common obstacles getting in the way of our transformation:

- *Time*
- *Guilt*
- *No energy*
- *Too confusing*
- *All or nothing*
- *Too overwhelming*

Let's talk some more about these things that get in our way when we want to move forward.

TIME

Time is far and away the most common objection we hear to taking action. If we had a pound for every time someone has said this to us, we'd be multi-millionaires.

"I don't have the time" "It will take too long" "I have to do this before I can do that" all of these and a few more I think you will recognise.

GUILT

Guilt is such a tough one because it's insidious. We so often put other peoples' needs before our own. That means we feel guilty when we're taking time for ourselves instead of using it for our employees, clients and family relying on us. We think that some of this stems from being a kid, seeing taking time off as some sort of luxury when everyone else is working. It's something that runs deep in a lot of people's blood as they don't want to appear selfish AND taking time for you... some think that's the epitome of being selfish.

ENERGY

What about **energy**? We can almost hear you agreeing with this one. How on earth are we supposed to find the energy to squeeze something else in when we're already feeling exhausted? It's the chicken and egg scenario. You don't have any energy because you're not doing anything, or it's because you're not doing anything that you don't have any energy? But the really good news is that doing this WILL create more energy.

CONFUSION

Confusion is a big deal. Starting something different causes us to want to rush back to do the same things we've done a million times expecting a different result. It's normal to be worried when you try something new but we've got the answer for you with our 4 S's, so read on.

ALL OR NOTHING

How many of us take the **'all or nothing'** approach in everything we do? We **overwhelm** ourselves and then throw the proverbial baby out with the bathwater when it's too much. The reason you might be in this pickle, like us, is because you are an overachiever, and someone who goes all in; however, we all know how that's ended up until now, right? Taking small, sustainable steps is the way to go. You can make one small change for a month and then add something else in. Darren Hardy, in his book 'The Compound Effect', says that it's the small things we do every day that lead to the biggest changes in our lives. He's right!

How many of these do you recognise? How many of these have you used? It's not just common in burn-out situations. It happens in a lot of areas of our lives. If you work in the service industry or have responsibility for staff, you'll recognise a few of these.

We want to help you give yourself the permission to move forward because you can't fill someone else's cup if your own is empty.

You will be better able to help your family, staff, colleagues and clients if you fill up your cup first.

Have a look at this cup. Is it full or is it empty? Is it useful? What is it? We all know the saying you can't pour from an E..... C..... . When we are depleted or knackered, we can't pour from our 'energy' cup if there is nothing in it.

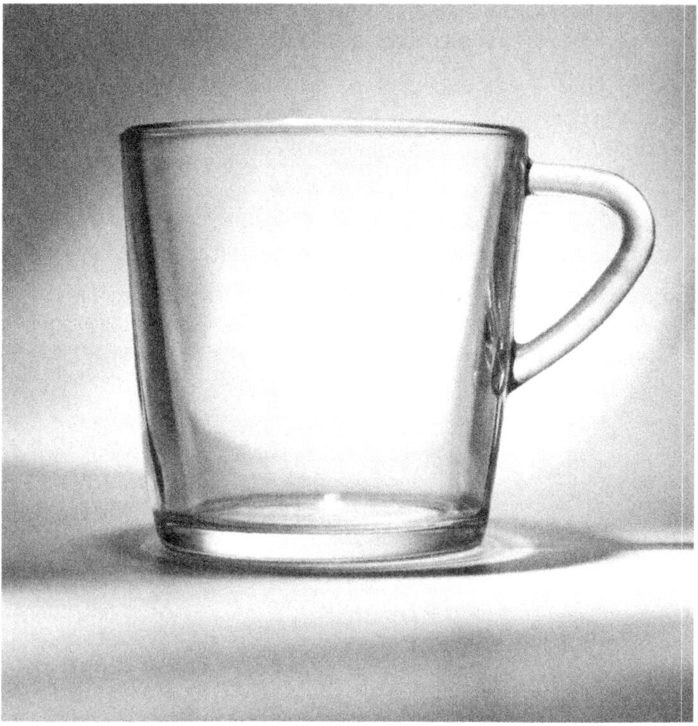

We've got to understand the truth of what we're doing here. Why are we looking after our health and wellbeing? Why are we focussed on getting out of burn-out? What is our intention behind all of this? It's all very well eating good food, doing exercise and getting sleep, but why? What is your overall intention? What are you trying to achieve?

This is something a lot of us don't think about. What's the intention of looking after ourselves? If you tell yourself 'I need to exercise' the objections will come thick and fast. Whereas if you set your intention to something different, then it changes again.

Here is an example. Loz goes to CrossFit three times a week and it takes three hours out of her day including the travel to and from the gym. If her intention is 'I'm going to CrossFit' then she feels really bad for leaving Baz to take care of everything else. But if she sets her intention to be 'by exercising I can shake up my energy to come back and give more quality time rather than quantity' then there is a different outcome. This she can justify.

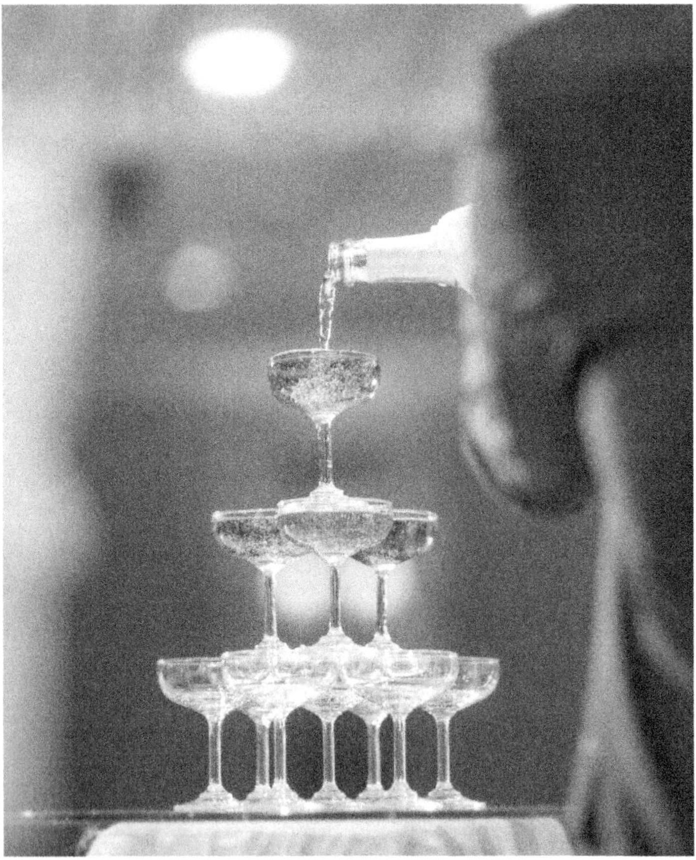

It comes back to the language you use. Why do you want to have an abundant lifestyle? Why did you set up your business in the first place? Why did you choose the work you do? And how are your actions going to help you achieve that outcome?

So what is this?

Okay, it's a fair guess that you got it right. It's a champagne tower. But what's happening here, metaphorically speaking?

Imagine you are the top glass in this tower and the champagne in it is the energy you are creating within you. Look at what is happening with that energy. Can you see what you're doing?

Imagine the glasses below are family members, colleagues, employees or clients. You are the person influencing their energy levels. You are the top of this hierarchy of energy.

Filling your glass up means it overflows and cascades down to the people below you, on to fill up the glasses of your closest level of family, business or clients. Then, as their cups also start to overflow, their extra energy flows down to the next level and so on. It creates a virtuous cycle of energy sharing and builds momentum. The more your cup overflows the more everyone in the tower of people below you will benefit.

However, if your glass is empty or dry, then they won't get anything. It does everyone around you a disservice not to share this positive energy you will be creating. But you need to create it first and that means giving yourself **permission** to do that.

As soon as you learn to create this energy and share it, the people around you are benefitting, and doing a service, to everyone in your world. All of the people around you are impacted by the energy you have. If you consider the benefit to them, then is the time taken to look after yourself really wasted?

We just love this picture because it just shows you how easily energy flows into and then out of our glass and into those below us. That energy is never going to be wasted because it will be used and replaced. Energy, and champagne, are meant to be used and replaced by new, fresh energy (and champagne).

This tower represents a celebration, as one of our clients pointed out to us in one of our sessions. We love the image even more since she said that.

People often ask us where we get our energy from because they see us as 'always on it'. Here is why. We have evenings and weekends off. Loz doesn't start work until 10am most days. We take holidays.

We always have energy because we look after ourselves. We do ALL of these things we're recommending to you guys. We surround ourselves with good and energetic people. We have invested in three coaches. We are always working on ourselves and investing in ourselves. The time and the money we've spent on ourselves has enabled us to be in this position. That's why we said at the beginning that it would be totally wrong for us to know all of this stuff having experienced its many benefits, and not share it with you.

THE DIFFERENCE BETWEEN ACTION AND INTENTIONAL ACTION

We really want to reiterate this so that we can help ensure you find taking action to be easy and fulfilling.

When we work with the guys on The Energised Leadership Program (which is our program helping you to tap into the flow to be able to create an abundant and healthy work-life balance and beating burn-out) we always encourage them to take INTENTIONAL action.

Intention is everything. So many just MAKE a plan or TAKE PART in a program. They just go through the motion mindlessly. It becomes a tick box exercise. Taking action in this way will 1. make you feel guilt for doing it when the going gets tough AND 2. ensure that the actions you take don't become part of your DNA.

New Year is a PRIME example. So many throw their arms in the air and say, "I want to lose 2 stone this year" so off they poodle DOING the 'thing', EATING the food, GOING to the gym, and when things get tough, they stop. WHY? because there was no intention behind it.

They are just invested in DOING the program AND NOT the transformation driven by the intention. If you want to take action and give yourself permission to make an impactful transformation, using intention is what you need to do. This is so often the level none of us think enough about. In the police force – there was no point just looking at the action, we needed to understand the intention or the motivation behind the action to solve a case, and to understand the offender.

DON'T JUST DO A PROGRAM INVEST THE TRANSFORMATION OF YOURSELF

So what is your intention or motivation behind this action? Is it coming from a place of guilt? Are you worried that the time spent on this action will be taken away from your business or career? That is what we call a low-level vibration. That is where your intention, the springboard for your action, is going to come from. Guilt and worry driving your intention are going to make it hard for you to move forward. Coming from that low-level vibration you'll be held down. It will feel like sandbags in a hot air balloon, preventing you from taking off towards your goal. You can see with this example how your intentions can change your vibrational energy and inevitably change the outcome.

Alternatively, your intention could be to give back and contribute, for example you could want to grow your business so you can help people. This could come from wanting to create a version of yourself that you truly want, deep in your heart. When you come from that intention the whole game changes. Every single day you can wake up and feel how achieving that will be for you. That will inspire you to take more action toward your goal.

- *Ask yourself these questions:*
- *What is the intention behind the outcome you want?*
- *Why is that goal important to you?*
- *Where does that intention come from?*

The energy you approach your action with affect the outcome. If you step up to the springboard to take a competition level dive fearful and expecting failure, the chances are that is exactly what will happen. But if you step up to it, confident and picturing yourself getting a perfect 10, then the chances are that's what you will achieve because your energy and intention are aligned.

What we really want you to do right now is to pick one thing intuitively that you believe will give you an instant boost of energy if you do it on a consistent basis.

Remember that your action needs to be simple, satisfying and sustainable. If its fun then that is even better.

Here are a few things that might work for you:

- *You might choose to adopt a morning or evening routine. You could tidy your bedroom; write out a to-do list; or take off your make-up before bed. Each of those things will make you feel good.*
- *Perhaps you could have a glass of water first thing in the morning, or swap one of your teas or coffees for water.*
- *You could set a timer to remind yourself that you need to drink more water during the day. You could even buy yourself a nice bottle to drink it from.*

- *You could plan your meals or even one of them.*
- *You could make some healthy swaps like salad instead of chips.*
- *You could simply take the time to sit down and have breakfast.*
- *You could do chair stretches at your desk.*
- *Or at lunch time you could take a short walk.*

All of these options are really simple things. The reason we're asking you to pick one is so that you can start taking action from that intention. So, changing your morning routine to include sitting down for breakfast could contribute to giving you more energy during the day, which means you will be able to help more people.

You can try and incorporate a couple of things but please don't overwhelm yourself. You don't need to do everything at once. Overwhelm is all about trying to do too much at once. Start something small, get into the habit doing that. Then once you've been doing it every day for one month, then you can add something else in. Each of these small, consistent steps are going to make a huge difference in 12months.

Give yourself permission and don't feel guilty. You owe it to the people who depend on you to take this action, even if you're unable to convince yourself that it's enough just to do it for your benefit.

Don't just DO the actions INVEST in a transformation of yourself on a deeper level through setting your intention.

THE REALITY OF TAKING ACTION

Taking action to manage your energy is critical to your business and career. Here are some of the reasons why:

- *It's part of your business strategy*
- *Your energy overflows into your business*
- *You have a duty of care to yourself and those working for you*
- *It will help achieve longevity in your business and career*
- *You're a role model, so teach by example*
- *It will make you and your team more resilient*

Let's consider some of these points a bit more.

If you own your business or look after staff, then this should be part of your **business or job role strategy**. What you put out in your workplace is ultimately going to affect your workplace and its output. It will overflow to your staff, your clients and impact the quality of your work.

It's actually your duty of care to consider your energy and wellbeing in relation to your business and workplace.

Let's consider an example. When we were in the police force and the prison service, we each had to pass a fitness test every single year. This was so that we would be fit enough to detain, chase, protect the perpetrators, manage prisoners, the public and our colleagues. It's a duty of care to the people you work with and for. Your mental and emotional health is a duty of care.

If we're not feeling 100%, we will cancel clients because our clients deserve 100% from us. We will respond to messages to us from clients acknowledging we've received their message and let them know that we will reply to them the next day when we can give them the energy and focus they deserve.

The reality is that taking action means you're going to have **longevity in your business and career**. There are so many people who face burn-out and this ends their careers. In Loz's case it took years but it caught up with her and she paid for it. What is the real cost of not taking a day off to re-energise or take some time out, or even a week to deal with burn-out, compared with having to leave a role or close your business because you've hit your big bang?

We've been running a business in the fitness industry for 8 years and our industry is known for being one of the most difficult to work in. We are here, showing up, with bundles of energy and we're not stopping.

All of us are **role models** in whatever business or work we do. We have to realise that others are learning through our example. To be a true leader you have to lead and you must lead by example. People will copy your behaviour. We developed a practice of 'checking in' and even known people who have long since left our world are still adopting that practice. We have taught them something incredibly valuable simply by showing them how it's done.

Taking actions to manage your energy makes you more **resilient**. When tough stuff comes your way and let's face it – that happens to all of us – none of us are immune to having difficult things in our lives. But by managing our energy and having an abundance of energy when we really need it, we make ourselves much more resilient. In practical terms it means that we don't get ill when we are under pressure. We have energy reserves that allow us to rise to the challenge when the pressure hits. That is what true resilience is.

How are you feeling about this information so far? Have you realised yet that this is bigger than you thought?

____

____

____

____

How do you take action?

Now you can see that you need to take intentional action but right now we bet you're asking yourself how to make it happen. There is so much to do.

However, this isn't something you will do in 90 days. It isn't something you will do in a week or two. This will take at least a year, and probably longer to achieve this. Because we cannot rush it. But there will be benefits and changes throughout that time as you stick to it.

Don't let the time to make real change put you off. We have a straightforward strategy to help you make it happen.

The 4 S's Ethos

To help you make these changes we have an Ethos called the '4 S's'. In simple terms whatever you do must be:

1. *Simple*
2. *Satisfying*
3. *Sustainable*
4. *and within a Supportive community*

When we talk about change being **simple,** we're referring to **progress over perfection**. We're not talking about committing to a programme, a meal plan or whatever other option comes up. We're talking about you committing to transforming your health, wellbeing and life. We always say keep it simple. If it's not simple then you're just not going to do it.

Satisfaction is the next part of our ethos. We need to ask ourselves – is this something I enjoy doing? Do I get a level of satisfaction from it? If you do then you will be prepared to do it again and again and again. How many times have you done something and walked away and realised how good it felt? You're already looking forward to going back and doing it again?

Repetition is the mother of all skills. So, when your action is satisfying you want to do it and therefore you will do it repeatedly. You'll never get slim by eating one salad. You'll never get overweight by eating one junk food meal. It's about finding something that fits your lifestyle that you can do every day and keep it up.

Any change you make must be **sustainable**. If you make it simple and satisfying then it will be sustainable. This is all about focusing on being consistent and persistent. It's also about educating yourself every day about how to challenge these habits and behaviours.

The last element is **support**. We are not saying you can't do this on your own because people can and do. But if you have the support or a community around you, you're going to be able to reach your goals much quicker. So many of the advantages of transformation come from support and community. They hold you in the space and help you to commit to moving forward. That is how you excel. That is the way to accelerate your transformation.

In our experience the people who really can do this all by themselves and achieve the same outcomes form a tiny, tiny percentage of the population. That's not because people aren't motivated, most of us are. However, that doesn't always translate into taking time out and prioritising what we need to do for ourselves.

Let's face it, most of the really successful people we know in our lives have coaches. They invest in people to encourage, mentor and advise them. In a lot of cases these coaches keep us accountable. The model works whether we're talking about business, health and wellbeing. Coaches move us forward, keep us accountable and hold our hands, especially when times get tough. When you invest in a coach what is really happening is you are buying speed, a quicker way to get what you want to achieve, with someone who's either been there or knows how to make it happen. When things are difficult, we so often revert back to what's easiest for us and what we're used to doing. But if we always do what we've always done, then the outcomes will always be the same as we've had before. For real change we need to push past that desire to go back to what we're used to and do what we haven't tried. The best way to do that is with support and community.

What actions should you take?

Now you know that taking action is not just about your wellbeing and energy management, it's also your duty of care for your businesses and jobs. You know that to transform your energy management you must make these actions simple, satisfying, sustainable and supportive. Now we're going to show what actions you should take in terms of the three dimensions of burn-out.

Here's a reminder:

- *Physical: Exhaustion*
- *Mental: Cynicism*
- *Emotional: Powerlessness*

Some of you may have ticked more for exhaustion and some for cynicism. Or you may relate more to the feelings around powerlessness. Maybe you've ticked all of them. It doesn't matter. This is all about looking at what action you can take. You don't need to take action on all of them at the same time. You might focus on one for a month and then another one for a month. This is about taking a journey that's nice and steady.

Let's take each of the three dimensions of burn-out and apply them to the six foundational pillars, identifying possible actions for you to take.

PHYSICAL: EXHAUSTION

Remember we discussed exhaustion, the physical side of burn-out, and how it relates to four of our foundational pillars – sleep, water, food and exercise. Look at some of the actions listed in our chart below. You'll see that they are all simple, satisfying, sustainable and you can get support for them.

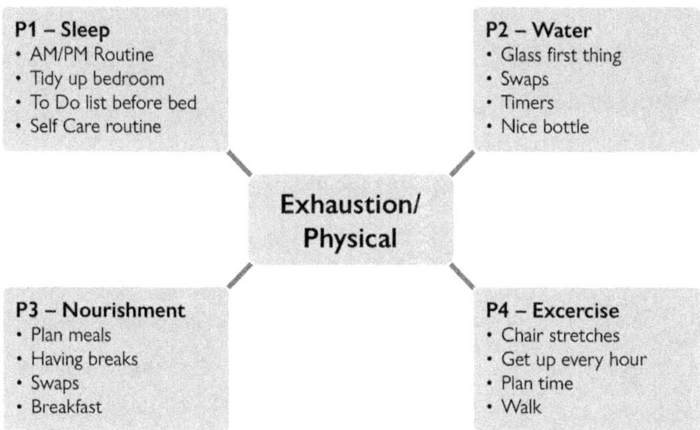

SLEEP

Let's consider sleep for a minute. How easy is it to set up a morning and evening routine so that you can sleep more easily? You don't have to do anything massive, sometimes just even

5-10 minutes will make a big difference?

Tidying up your bedroom will provide an uncluttered space for your brain and body to rest better. If you do it every morning it won't take more than five minutes a day. It won't be an epic, exhausting effort every week or fortnight that feels overwhelming and exhausting.

Before you go to bed you can do a to-do list for the next day so you can go to sleep knowing that you have a plan for the next day.

Or you could set up a self-care routine where you wash the day off with a shower? Or take your make-up off (for men and ladies) and do a lovely skin care routine?

All of these things are really simple. We're not talking about massive actions that will turn your life upside down.

We are talking about small steps in order to get you to where you need to go.

Remember you only need to start with one. Do that for a month and then perhaps add another one.

WATER

Just having one glass first thing in the morning is just one example of an easy thing you can do to get a great start on your day.

Swap a couple of your cups of tea and coffee for water.

Set a timer to remind yourself that you need to drink, it's so easy to forget when you're busy. Most of us can set alarms on our phones but there are some fancy water bottles that have timers with them.

You could even get yourself a beautiful water bottle that

makes you want to drink out of them. We've both got snazzy water bottles. Loz has crystals in hers and both of ours are made of glass rather than plastic. These really simple things, done every day, will make such a big difference.

FOOD

One option that is easy to make happen is to plan your meals and take breaks. How much nicer would that be than swallowing a hasty sandwich you hardly taste while you're working at your computer. The other thing to note about this is that when we sit and take 5-10 minutes to actually eat our food, we eat it mindfully. It also allows our digestive system to concentrate on what it's meant to do...digest our food.

9 times out of 10 we are running about doing everything all at once, it causes our autonomic nervous system to be in fight or flight rather than rest and digest. When you sit down and eat your food in peace you will avoid the bloating, and the acid indigestion many people face after eating.

Swap some of your sandwiches for fresh, healthy, tasty salads with loads of bright coloured salad leaves, tomatoes, cucumbers and peppers in them. Sit, enjoy the time and savour the taste and texture.

Breakfast is such a great way to give you energy to start your day. Porridge is easy and quick to make. But again, more importantly, make this part of your morning routine. Take the time to sit and gather yourself for 5 minutes before you rush out of the door. In some religions they actually taketime to bless their food. Essentially what they are doing is lifting their whole spirit mentally, emotionally, spiritually and physically too, all through just taking a few moments to be thankful for what is in front of them and how it is going to nourish them.

Healthy eating is just about making a few different choices. We all need to eat and we all pretty much eat three meals a day. So, when it comes to mealtime just think about what you're going to eat. When it comes to eating, just ask yourself "Is this the healthiest choice for me right now that will nourish my body with the fuel I need to manage my energy?"

Imagine the pleasure of a healthy, fresh, simple meal when you're tired and need an injection of energy, rather than something quick that might make you feel (even more) sluggish and tired.

EXERCISE

Exercise is really about movement. You don't have to think about exercise as a big thing. There are so many small things we can do that will make a huge difference if we do them every day. Chair stretches and getting up and moving around for a few minutes every hour that you work, are such easy ways of looking after our bodies, and the bonus is you'll get less aches and pains. Having a short walk at lunch time and even wandering in a park or garden for a few minutes are all small but helpful activities.

While we were working on this book we worked for an hour and a half and Loz got up and went outside into the garden to plant her feet into the dirt for five or ten minutes. After that she felt refreshed and got straight back into writing. Because she'd taken those few minutes out in the garden, she produced quality work rather than just a lot of it. We all know that it's quality not quantity work we want to put out.

All of the actions above compound over time make huge differences. We know this because we do them every single day.

MENTAL: CYNICISM

If you resonate with cynicism then this is all about your mind. It's about making sure our brains are not overwhelmed and that's why it falls under pillar five which is about thought management.

Pillar 5 – Thought Management

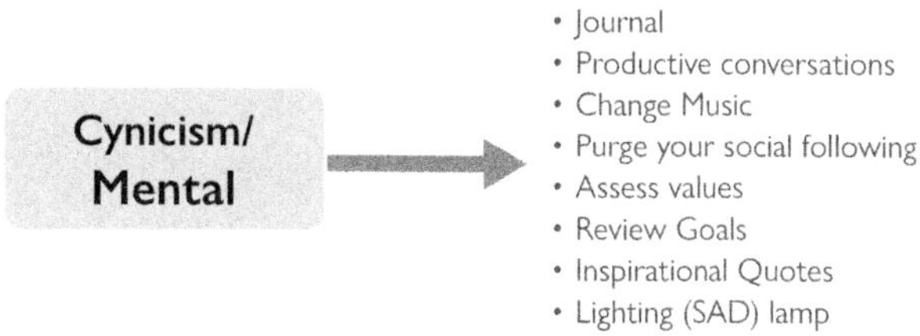

THOUGHT MANAGEMENT

There are so many easy ways to deal with being in a state of overwhelm. These are just a few very simple ways to do that.

Journaling is such an easy and effective thing to do. It clears your head so that you are more productive and can focus on your work and life more easily. There are no rules with journaling but even ten minutes every morning or evening can make a huge difference. Another thing that you could choose to add to your journaling is adding the things that you're grateful for. Some people suggest listing three things that you are happy about. It can be as simple as:

'I am grateful for the safe and warm home I live in.'

'I am grateful for a full fridge.'

'I'm grateful I have enough money to pay my rent.'

It helps give us perspective and reminds us that some people don't have a safe or warm home, a full fridge or money to pay rent.

There are some who suggest that this simple exercise can, in fact, attract more abundance into our lives to be grateful for.

And it's so simple and quick!

There have actually been clinical studies into this and they have proven that journaling can improve depression symptoms simply by doing just 5 minutes over 2-3 days per week. ([4]Another option is having productive conversations. Who are you talking to? Have a conversation with someone. It could stimulate you or make you laugh, or even put your life into a bit of perspective. Sometimes our brain enjoys the break from what it's usually engaged in thinking about.

Change the music you're listening to. Music has such a way of changing our moods. In college Baz and his mates did an experiment. They tested their heart rate while they listened to different types of music. They found their heart rate was changing depending on what they listened to. This tiny difference can change how you think and feel. Just look up "happy" playlist and see what comes up. Even if it gets your shoulders shimmying for a little bit, it's all doing the same thing.

Purging your social media followers can make a difference. Are their posts or comments filling your cup up or are they feeding any feelings of cynicism you're experiencing? We all have a responsibility to know what is happening in the world around us but if you're suffering burn-out then do you need to know about whatever they're posting right now? Don't be scared to block or mute them. It's your feed, you can do what you want. You can mute people without them having any idea you've done it. Or even snooze them for a while, until you feel better.

Inspirational quotes are another great option. They do just that – they inspire us! Loz looks at them every day and then shares them with Baz. Every now and then they are just perfect for the mood or space we find ourselves in.

A big one that works in our lives is a SAD lamp. We've got one in our office and when we're feeling really low in energy, we flick it on and boom our energy raises! So many of us lack vitamin D and these lamps can really help to boost our energy, mood, sleep and reduce depression.

GREAT TIP:

One exercise that you can use that will definitely help is to assess your values.

What are your values in your life and which ones are most important? In the hierarchy of what is most significant, which values are at the top? If something is at the top of your list then you're going to invest more to achieve that. Have a little look at them.

Review your goals. What is it you want out of life? If you really want something you're going to push towards it. Does an action further your goals? If so, that will be a real motivator to making these small changes.

You can use your journaling to assess your values and to review your goals. When we're exhausted, we tend to lose sight of our purpose or we question it because nothing feels as motivating or exciting as it did when we had more energy.

One of the implications of this is that you can find that your clients no longer fit your goals or purpose. If working with them doesn't feel right or is emptying your cup more than the amount that is taken just from the work itself then refer them on. They could be someone else's dream client. If you're not gelling it's probably not working for them either and there's a strong chance, they won't be getting the results they want.

When our values do not align with our behaviour, we can feel an icky friction that doesn't sit right with us. It can have you up at all hours and if you're not aligned you won't be able to do much. This is what is usually happening with this phase.

None of us like to think of ourselves as a negative Nelly, or a judgemental Judy but it happens.

> *'I know for me that this was a huge one. I had not defined my version of success and was looking at everyone else's goals and had forgotten my own. No wonder I went BANG when I was trying to pin my happiness on someone else's goals and success. It does not happen.'* **Loz**

EMOTIONAL: POWERLESSNESS

The final dimension we want to discuss is about powerlessness, which relates to the emotions of burn-out. Not feeling good enough is a big part of this. It fits in with our pillar 6 which is DeStress Me Time.

Pillar 6 – DeStressMeTime

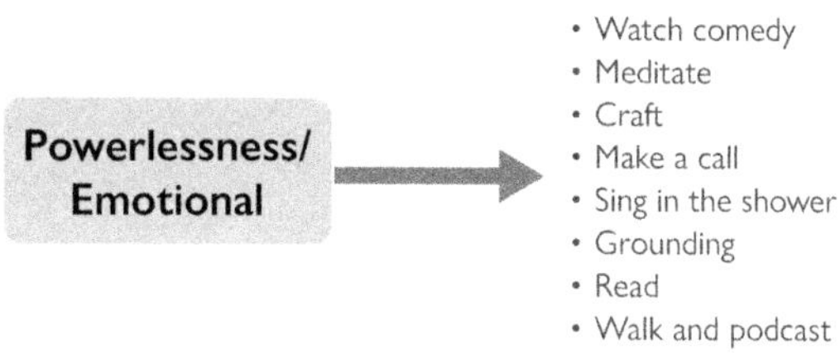

DeStress Me Time

> *'This is a really important one for me. Burn-out starts showing up for me as not feeling good enough, because I was chasing someone else's idea of success and happiness, and the dreaded imposter syndrome kicked in. So, I keep doing simple things like this to keep me on top of it.'* **Loz**

Burn-out symptoms, especially if they're long running can feel a lot like a mental or chronic illness. Doing simple things every day can keep them at bay. Mastery is about doing things on a daily basis.

'You have to do these things every day, to keep burn-out at bay'.

Some really simple and fun things you can do include watching comedy. Even if you don't laugh out loud and it just makes you smile or giggle inside, then it's done its job.

> *'Michael McIntyre got me through some of my darkest days. I also love the Cookie Monster being a life coach – its's pure gold!'* **Loz**

Meditation, art & craft work, singing in the shower, going outside and putting your feet in dirt are all great options and the joy is that you don't have to be good at any of these things – you can just do them for yourself. Read a great book, listen to an inspiring or entertaining podcast or just go for a walk.

I'm sure you can see that all of these things are very, very simple things to do and ...well...fun. They don't take up much time but they will make you feel better, lighter and happier. They'll give you a level of satisfaction and because they are both simple and satisfying, that will make them sustainable especially if you have a supportive network or community.

How is this sitting with you right now? Take stock of what you've read and think about what feels good to you.

____

____

____

____

Remember all of this is just about filling up your cup so that it can overflow and share your energy with others. That's all we're doing here. These are the simple, satisfying ways to become a rock solid, abundant leader. Filling up your cup so it overflows with abundance and benefits all of those around you is just the way to do it.

How would it feel if someone walked into your office and felt your energy? It's that energy that attracts abundance to you. People buy into people, they buy your energy. So, if you're in the business of selling or providing a service or product, clients are going to buy into you, into your energy and what you're giving off.

You know yourself that when you walk into a room you can feel the energy a person is giving off whether it's positive or negative. That's just another advantage to taking the time to fill your energy cup.

How do we turn these actions into habits? Let's talk about that now.

HABIT CREATION

We want to deal with burn-out, get out from under it. To do that we need to create some habits so it doesn't happen again and so we can attract health, wealth and abundance. We can live the life we want to live.

How long do you think it takes for people to build a habit?

We've all seen studies that have suggested that creating a habit takes from 18 days to 254 days. So, that range runs from a bit more than two weeks to just under a year. You've probably heard the most common opinion, that it takes 21 days. Given the lack of agreement on how long it takes, let's concentrate on how to effectively create a habit.

HOW DO YOU FORM A HABIT?

Let's think about a habit we've all formed. How many of you remember learning to brush your teeth every day? What happened? How did you form that habit?

You didn't just get up at four or five years old and decide to brush your teeth. It was probably the last thing on your mind. You didn't get up and just do it yourself. You had support, probably from your parents, who constantly reminded you every single day, twice a day. Your parents were supporting you and coaching you to do this.

How long does it take to form a habit exactly? Well, a study conducted by Philippa Lally who is a health psychology researcher at University College London investigated this.

This study was published in the European Journal of Social Psychology. Lally and her team's aim was to figure out how long it takes to form a habit.

Over a 12-week period they examined the habits of 96 people. Each of the participants chose one new habit for that 12-week period and each day they had to report on whether they did their new chosen behaviour or not and in addition how "automatic" it felt.

The type of habits that were chosen varied from drinking a bottle of water with lunch or running 15 minutes before dinner.

At the end of the 12 weeks, the researchers reviewed the data to see how long it took each person to go from starting a new behaviour to automatically doing it.

What did they find? Well, it's not exactly a surprise. It was found that on average, it can take more than 2 months before a new behaviour becomes "automatic". The sweet spot was 66 days to be precise.

But they also found some nuisances. What they found what that how long it takes to form a new habit can really deepens on A. The behaviour, B. The person and C. The circumstance

In the study itself they found it took anywhere from 18 days to 254 days for people to form a new habit.

To really make your new habit stick takes effort and reminders everyday and to surround yourself with people who will encourage, remind or coach you to continue. You can start something and get into the habit of it but how do you commit to it? How do you make sure you'll still be doing it five years from now?

It doesn't matter what you want to master, mastery requires dedicated, daily habits over the long term.

Think about martial arts – karate or judo, for example. We associate those who are good at martial arts as masters. Why are they masters? Because they practice the fundamentals every single day, for example Katas. They practice movement patterns every day so they don't have to think about them. That is the true art of mastery – when they become second nature and we don't have to think about them. They become automatic and save you energy.

So, how are you going to give yourself the permission to take one satisfying action towards building your energy and filling your cup up?

There is a fabulous book called 'Atomic Habits' by James Clear which talks about creating new habits and breaking old ones. It's brilliant for this.

Let's move on to The Focus.

CHAPTER SIX

The Focus

The future belongs to those who believe in the beauty of their dreams

---

Eleanor Roosevelt

In the last chapter we dealt with the tricky issue of giving ourselves permission to take time for ourselves to transform our energy management. Step 4 is about The Focus. This is the bit where we **assess and adjust our actions**. We call it the YOU strategy. This chapter is really important, especially if you're a stop/starter.

- *We're going to look at these issues:*
- *The reasons people stop*
- *Strategy in your business*
- *Cycles of energy and change*
- *Blueprint for assessing and adjusting what's right under your nose*

Strategies

Let's talk about strategies. Just think for a moment about your business and career. Whatever it is you do you will have strategies in place. They are likely to include:

- *Marketing*
- *Cash flow*
- *Social media*
- *Sales*
- *Employees*
- *Copywriting*

- *Retention*
- *System and processes*

If you're in a business or in a senior role just think for a minute about how many of these or other strategies you have in place.

____

____

____

____

How often do you assess and adjust these? In our business we are always working on marketing. We think about our social media and assess what images or copy landed well and how they might be better. We're constantly looking at analytics to see what social media has worked best for our business. This is how we keep our business moving forward.

You should always be assessing your sales, cash flow and other strategies to make sure they're working for you and that you're moving in the right direction. And, if they're not, then they need adjusting.

When you have strategies in your business you need to keep developing them and constantly learning and updating them. Nine times out of ten people will put in place strategies that others have used. They assume that's the way it's done and that it will work for them. However, we often need to take a step back and first consider what we need to put in place for ourselves and our business. Every business is not the same and there are no 'one size fits all' options that will work for everyone.

We're sure you're nodding your head right now. So, having said that, what are your strategies for keeping healthy and managing your energy? More importantly – do you assess those strategies? Or do you just put them in place and decide that's what you're doing and that's how it will be from now on? Or do you take time to step back and look at what is happening and how it's working? Do you just do what other people are doing without deciding first whether they will work for you? Nothing stays the same, everything changes.

We all know that to have a successful business/career we need all of the strategies above - looking after ourselves is no different. All of the successful people we know have these strategies in place. Their strategies will be adapted and adjusted, but there is one constant, they are always in place.

How many times have you started a health regimen only to stop when the food you are meant to be eating was not on the menu, or you couldn't fit in the workout because you had other commitments. You more than likely just said "I'll start again Monday" but that Monday never comes. If that's you then THIS is going to be crucial to you stopping the hamster wheel of 'off and on'.

So, stop here for a minute. If you haven't already done so, ask yourself why you have stopped in the past.

Did you ever take the time to ask yourself these questions?

- *Is this working for me?*
- *How can I improve this?*

Or did you just stop?

'The quality of your life depends on the quality of your questions.' **Tony Robbins**

You can either ask yourself stagnation questions or you can ask yourself propulsion questions.

Stagnation questions are why am I always burned out? Why is this happening to me? Why am I so useless?

Propulsion questions are how can I make this better? What am I seeing right now? How can I do this and have fun? What's the best way for me to deal with burn-out?

It's time to put some strategies into place for your health that you have in place for your business. Here are some of the questions you can ask yourself to assess and adjust your strategies. We recommend doing this every 6-8 weeks. Ask yourself questions like these:

- *Is this working for me?*
- *How can I improve this?*
- *Was it simple?*
- *Is this filling or emptying my cup?*
- *What type of energy is this?*

Rather than asking yourself why this isn't working for you? And telling yourself this is never going to work.

There is a very different energy in the questions you're asking yourself with these ones.

How to assess and adjust

We have developed a 4-step process for you to assess your strategies and decide if anything needs adjusting. This process plays out in every single module on our Energised Leadership Program because we don't just want you to do this once. Remember this is all about transformation.

When you come up against a struggle or you notice that you have stopped doing your intentional action, take some time and use this model to help you to adjust your strategy and get right back to it.

Step One: Accept and acknowledge (The Space)

In this step ask yourself:

What have I acknowledged about this situation?

What have I accepted about this situation?

What am I seeing that wasn't there before?

Step Two: Create Awareness (The Insight)

What would happen if I changed this?

Could I make this better or more effective?

What has changed recently?

Is this serving me anymore? (If yes, how? If no, why not?)

Am I just doing this thing (going through the motions) or am I intentionally transforming?

What am I seeing now that wasn't there before?

Step Three: Taking Action (The Permission)

How will this positively impact me?

What is one simple and effective change I could make right now?

How can I implement this?

Step Four: Accelerate (The Connection)

Do I need any help with this?

If yes, what help do I need? And who can help me?

What will I do to make sure I get the help I need?

____

____

____

____

____

This 4-step process will help you uncover what you need to adjust and how. Remember that key to making any lasting adjustments is that you must give them time to work. One session at the gym isn't going to make a change, one salad isn't going to help you lose weight, one glass of water on only one morning isn't going to make a sustainable difference. If it did, we would all be millionaires!

Now let's talk about how we know when to assess and adjust.

- *There are 3 occasions when you might want to assess and adjust:*
- *Internal feelings*
- *External influences*
- *Situational Changes*

Internally, thanks to our intuition we assess and adjust regularly and frequently. In fact, we do that as much as twice in a second. Our intuition is what we call our Spidey-sense. It's that message or feeling of discomfort deep in our gut that something isn't quite right. Most of us have learned the hard way that ignoring that feeling is a very bad idea. This is a reality for so many of us because we're so busy and have too much noise going around in our heads, so we ignore the signs about what's really happening.

Stop and work out what it's trying to tell you. You will get external and internal "spidey-sense" feelings around this.

Internal feelings will be things going on inside of you that your intuition or gut feels and this can come up at any time. That is why it's so important to know about the 3 dimensions of burn-out and the signs and symptoms and know this stuff inside out and back to front. It could be for you when you feel like you've lost your enthusiasm for what you do. Perhaps you've been passionate about it but all of a sudden, it's lost its sparkle. What if you're starting to feel tired and just not feeling quite like yourself? It could be that a simple tweak to your daily routine can put that sparkle back?

One thing that works really well in terms of internal assessments is to write on a piece of paper. It connects us to our subconscious effectively. Just write for five or ten minutes and put on your 'detective specs'. Ask what is happening here? What has changed? Why am I feeling like this? In time, your intuition will let you know when something needs adjusting, just make sure you are listening to it.

In terms of our external assessment and adjustment here we recommend assessing every three to six months. Just a brief assessment of everything you're doing – food, exercise, business, diary, finances, marketing, tweaking as you go.

Additionally, you might just want to check in on things when something significant changes:

- *Have you got a new, big client?*
- *Have you noticed a reduction in clients?*
- *Do you need more people in your team?*
- *Are you doing too many hours at work?*
- *Are you noticing that you are more fatigued?*
- *Are your work clothes tighter?*
- *Have your personal circumstances changed? Children, school, study, relationships?*

When something changes in your life or at work it's a great time to take stock and see if anything needs adjusting.

Before and after holidays are a great time to assess whether you are feeling fit and healthy. Sometimes we just need a break but if that doesn't work as well as you'd like, perhaps you need to assess whether you are getting enough sleep.

Christmas and the New Year are a good time to assess health related issues. It's flu season so if you've not been looking after yourself then the effects are more likely to show up then.

WHY DO PEOPLE STOP?

Let's talk about the elephant in the room – sometimes people stop putting into practice their chosen actions. So, let's list some of the reasons people tend to stop. This can be because:

- *We think it's not working and/or we've reached a plateau because progress seems to stop or slow down;*
- *We get bored doing the same thing or eating the same things and we need to change our thinking around them;*
- *We haven't got a coach or someone to hold us accountable or to remind us of what we need to be doing, and why, on a regular basis;*
- *We put ourselves last. Everyone else's needs are more important than ours.*

In so many cases it's because you've hit a plateau. Things have started slowing down or you've stopped. Nine times out of ten in response to this we become a digger or a climber. That can be construed as having reached our goal; or we've reached an obstacle that we can't find a way around or over.

A digger is likely to reach a plateau and just keep digging. They will see the plateau as a failure and keep doing the same thing over and over again, getting deeper and deeper into their hole.

Climbers get excited about a plateau. They look up and use it as an opportunity to climb higher. They seek advice from people who have been there and done what they want to achieve. They keep going forward and they relish it.

Things do change and will change if we have the right approach.

Sometimes all we need to do is to take different action or approach to resolve these things.

We spoke about setting a habit in motion and that requires us to do the same thing over and over again. Sometimes we get bored having to do the same thing day in-day out but here's the thing.

'There's magic in the mundane'

There's nothing sexy about drinking water. There's nothing sexy about eating food, going to bed and getting up and doing it all again the next day. The problem is that we get bored because we miss the magic in the mundane.

The other thing that can happen is that we wander off our path. We can lose sight of our purpose. We know every single day what our purpose is. We know what it is we're here to do on this planet. We know what we're working towards and we don't forget that. When we do get a bit 'over it' and find ourselves fed up doing the same thing every day we need to remind ourselves what our purpose is.

Of course, if you are feeling the cynicism or powerlessness of burn-out, that can definitely influence people to stop.

But let us remind you again that things will change and do change.

> *'When I left the police service the strategy I'd had as an entrepreneur didn't work for me at all. It wasn't working but I'd had in my head that this was the way it was meant to be done, so I kept doing the same thing. Then things got much busier, we got a lot more clients so we started playing a bigger game. I had to change how I dealt with my mental health yet again.'* **Loz**

Now we are stepping up again doing this type of training and working with corporations. Things have to change. Nothing stays the same and once you've grasped that then you know that you have to have strategies for your health, in the same way you do for your business.

Remember earlier in the book we talked about water. Water is constantly moving, constantly in flow, constantly adapting to the environment around it. As soon as that water stops it becomes stagnant and toxic and that's what we cannot allow our energy to do. We can't let it become that way so we have to keep letting our energy flow.

That leads us nicely on to the next part which is about energy cycles.

ENERGY CYCLES

All energies are on a cycle of change, they are cyclical. Think of all of these:

- *The seasons*
- *Sun and the moon*
- *Weather*

- *Menstruation*
- *Fashion*
- *Weeks/Days*
- *Time*

They are all cycles of energy. Nearly everything that governs us and our lives is some sort of energy cycle.

What we don't really think about is how we adjust around those cycles. The seasons and weather are great examples. We don't realise that we adjust what we wear according to the seasons, because we've been doing it for so long. We don't tend to wear scarves and jumpers in summer or swimsuits in winter. At some level we're constantly assessing and adjusting our behaviour. We don't stick to wearing our tank tops when the weather is freezing because that's what we'd decided to do – we adapt to the change in conditions. We consider the 'new conditions' and put a jumper or leggings on.

If you look at the magic of mundane, you're going to have some times when you are just doing some of the simple, easy, boring stuff like drinking the water, going to bed, eating your breakfast, doing your journaling and it might feel like it's going nowhere. But let's look at a tree and the seasons as an example. A tree might look dead in winter – like it's doing nothing. Underneath what you can't see is that tree preparing itself for new growth, then loss of its leaves and back to winter. You can't see what it is doing but it is preparing itself and doing what it needs to do right now to grow and bloom at the right time. To be ready when we need to be at our best, we need to keep burn-out at bay so we must do the same and work within our energy cycles.

It doesn't make sense to think that you'll take the same approach every day regardless of what is happening around you. The same approach is not going to work in every season, in every part of the year, in every economic cycle or, as we have seen throughout Covid, during the completely unexpected. If people had already been facing burn-out before Covid, their capacity to adjust in a period where so much adaptation was required would have felt too much. They would have had no reserves to deal with that on top of everything else. It has been difficult enough to deal without trying to apply the old approach to a new situation.

Our energy has cycles. We have periods of high and low energy and it's about managing them. When we are in a low energy or mood cycle and feeling bored or dissatisfied our job is just to keep moving forward.

There's a time for go and a time for slow.

So many people ask us for a blueprint for success. What we really want to make clear here is that you already have that blueprint. All of those areas you've succeeded so well in show that you already have strategies that are working. The trick is to use what you already have, what you already know, alongside the information in this book to apply that to the aspects of your life you're not 100% happy with.

If you're feeling like it would help then we're going to share an exercise we use with our one-to-one and corporate clients. It's called the Wheel of Life. It might seem a bit of a no-brainer as an exercise but as simple as it looks, we've all been surprised at what it can reveal.

It will help you see very visually the areas of your life where you've really succeeded and will help you decipher why you're so successful in certain areas and not so much in other areas. You can find this strategy at the back of this book. We really hope it helps.

This is one of the reasons we talk about people immediately taking action before they take these steps. If you're taking action, especially when you're struggling with burn-out how can you know that you're taking the right action for the right results? Each of these steps are critical to the success and sustainability of managing your energy.

The next step, The Connection, is the icing on the cake and will make sure you get to where you want to faster.

CHAPTER SEVEN

The Connection

A connection is the feeling you get when you're with someone. It's not just a physical connection, but an emotional one

---

Anon

We love step 5 of our energy reset programme because it's the icing on the cake.

By the time we get to this point in the programme we are always so energised. We think that once you get to this point – once you master your energy then you master your life.

This step is all about **The Connection and Acceleration.**

Before we move on to this step. Take a few minutes to think about what you've learned so far. What are your top takeaways from the first four steps?

___

___

___

___

___

Have you had a lightbulb moment?

What is the biggest thing you've taken away from this book so far?

In this step we're going to cover:

- *The Missing Piece*
- *What usually happens when you don't have this?*

- *How to become a master of your energy*
- *The greats and how they're successful*
- *The icing on the cake – the Connection*
- *The importance of a support network and coaching*

THE MISSING PIECE

The missing piece is about the people, support and community around you to help you move forward in transforming your energy management.

Here are a few questions for you to consider before we move on:

- *Do you have people around you who support you?*
- *Do you have people in your life who won't let you off with excuses?*
- *Are there people around you who will lift you up?*
- *Do you have people who will support your dreams/ goals?*
- *Are you around people who can develop you – in business, career, mentally, emotionally, spiritually and physically?*

We need to surround ourselves with certain types of people who can help us on this journey. We've all heard the quote 'Birds of a feather, flock together'. You never see a flock of magpies with an eagle in their midst. We all want to be around people who can help us be who we want to be.

Sometimes people simply need to remind us of what we already know and what our reasons were for getting started in the first place. We can so easily lose sight of these things with everything going on in our brains.

You need to sit back and ask all of these questions. Then answer them honestly. Don't worry if you discover there aren't people around who support you or who question your excuses for not acting or sticking with it. It's okay to admit that. If they aren't in your life right now then they can be. There are people out there who will do that for you, and you can do that for them as well.

- *When we're overwhelmed or stressed, we can find ourselves doing one or more of these:*
- *Distancing ourselves*
- *Putting our head down and just working*
- *Isolating ourselves*
- *Suffering in silence*
- *Not asking for help*
- *Feeling stuck and lost*
- *Feeling like we're in a dark place*
- *Stagnating and festering*

The first thing we do is **distance ourselves**. We lock ourselves away. Then we **put our head in our work** as an effective distraction so we don't have to think about what we're overwhelmed by. We just concentrate on our work. We think that if we keep doing the work then we might push ourselves through and come out the other side. We can assure you that that doesn't happen. The problem doesn't just go away or resolve itself because we're not thinking about it. **We isolate ourselves** from those around us or the things we want to do.

Suffering in silence is a big one. A lot of guys come to us and they don't speak up. Inside they are beating themselves up and they don't talk to anyone about it. We need to talk about these things and to share how we're feeling.

This moves us on to the next point which is that **people don't ask for help**. Everyone needs help sometimes. Even those of you at the very top of your game need to ask for help.

Feeling **stuck and lost** is a tough one. It's tempting to do nothing, to sit and twiddle your thumbs in the hope that something will change if you just wait for it but it doesn't. That can be a really **dark place** to be in and connects back to suffering in silence. The result is that you just **stagnate and fester** in it.

If you surround yourself with people who are in the same place and none of the people around you are taking action or assessing how to move forward then you'll all fester in that energy together. Relating to each other is one thing and that can be really helpful but once you've acknowledged and identified the problem you need to be able to move forward and that's not going to happen if you're surrounded by people who are stuck and not in any hurry to do anything to shift their energy or strategy.

Remember birds of like feather flock together

Some self-help groups can be a bit like this. Once they've provided a safe space for people to relate and resonate with each other, they don't have a way to help people shift forward and to find different approaches that work for their community. Of course, some do and they can be really powerful if people can see others moving forward and finding ways around the obstacles they face rather than staying stuck.

Do you recognise any of these points? Have you felt like this? Is this what happens to you? Which ones do you relate to and why? How does it feel when you find yourself there?

____

____

____

____

This stagnant, toxic energy can keep you stuck in a dark place for days, weeks or even years if you don't do something different.

You know the formula to becoming a master of your energy

- *You know the 4 steps up to this point – we've been covering them since the beginning of this book*
- *You know that you need to practice it*
- *You know deep inside that you need to take you time, be easy on yourself and not try to do it all at once*
- *You know that you need to use the 4 S's – simple, satisfying, sustainable and supportive*
- *You know that we need to have a mission, a purpose, a 'why'*

The problem is that we don't do it. This is the power of connection.

Let's look at some successful people and think about what they do. What is it about successful people like:

- *Richard Branson*
- *Michelle Obama*
- *Sylvester Stallone*
- *JLo (Jennifer Lopez)*
- *The Rock (Dwayne Johnson); and*
- *Tony Robbins*

Why have they succeeded where others in the same fields haven't?

Richard Branson has run highly successful businesses and is well known the world over. He's not without his challenges but he hasn't let them stop him. Michelle Obama is brilliant and successful in a world where being black and a woman has not been an advantage. She is an influencer on global issues. You get the picture. Each of the people in this list, and many others have reached the top of the heap in what are very competitive areas. There are no doubt many, many others you can think of.

What successful people have in common is that they have coaches and advisors. People who are invested in them achieving their missions.

In our lives and business, we like to spend time with people who have a higher energy or a higher vibration than us. We like to be around people who are more successful than us because then it will rub off on us. The other thing you've got to remember if you're in business or you have a career, 9 times out of 10 much of your help and advice comes from your network, the people around you. We can't underestimate the value of a solid network.

All of the successful people above are where they are because they've employed coaches to get them to the next step, they've built connections with people who are successful in their own areas and that knowledge, experience and network has helped them and can help us. These connections can help us get to the next level. We don't know many people who have achieved enormous success in any area of their lives, that have done it on their own.

Everyone who has been successful has people behind them who have helped them on their way. We've thought about this and we can't think of a single successful person who has done it on their own.

Even superheroes need someone to help them out, none of them can do it by themselves and they have superpowers! Even Batman needed Alfred and Robin.

We don't just mean people who are successful in business and in corporate life by the way, we mean people who are successful in life. Oprah, for example, mastered meditation because of Deepak Chopra. Tony Robbins employed a coach, Jim Rohn. They've found the best in the business and sought them out to get advice and coaching from them. We happen to know quite a bit about Sylvester Stallone because one of our mentors Rehan Jalali is his coach. He knows the struggles Sylvester Stallone has had and the people and connections he's needed to use to help him get where he is today. He didn't just start out looking amazing in Rocky – Rehan actually helped him to look as fit as he did.

Of course, we recommend looking for people who have managed to address all of the areas of their lives. We think you can only be as successful as you can be if your health – both mental and physical - is as good as it can be. Oprah would've needed a lot of business-related advice and coaching but she recognised a need for balance in her life and got help from Deepak Chopra to meditate.

Anyone can be a success in one area of their lives but if they ignore everything else and their health crashes, it will directly impact their business and career, and their family life.

The connections you need are decided by the values and your mission in life. If one of your priorities in life is getting healthy and mastering your energy you wouldn't go to Richard Branson or Alan Sugar for that. If you wanted help running your business you wouldn't choose The Rock for advice. The help you look for is based on the priority areas you want to develop in your life. The areas you want to raise to higher levels on your Wheel of Life.

Richard Branson has had some enormous fails. Not too long ago a man died because of an epic failing while sending one of his rockets into space. However, the way he dealt with that was to ask people for help to get through that period. Getting through that terrible time would've been impossible by himself.

All of our efforts are not going to be huge successes but it's much more likely to be a success if you ask the right people for help. We need people to help us move forward and to pick us up when we fall. That's so powerful because if you have that in place, you'll be much less afraid of moving forward and you won't let fear get in the way of acting.

It makes sense that the icing on the cake **is that connection.** Connection **being** the 'state of being related to someone or something else'.[5]

It's claimed that you are the sum of the 5 people you hang about with most online or in person. We think that this is true. Energy is transferable both online and in person. Think of a movie where someone gets frightened and it affects everyone else. Other people can 'catch' energy from others – both positive and negative.

Think about a bowl of fruit where one piece is mouldy. If you leave that mouldy piece of fruit in the bowl then all of the others will get mouldy too. One bad, mouldy apple can cause the rest of the apples to go mouldy because ethylene gas that causes the fruit to ripen is to blame.

Here's the thing – we know the power of this. We absolutely know the power of connection, community and support. We are so proud of the people we have in our world and the communities we have, where we have brought people together because it really takes something special to bring a bunch of people together and get them working in a connective way. One of the things we are most proud of and feel comfortable bragging about is literally the powerful community that we have. They are amazing people. So, we know the power of that network – if someone is down, someone else will pick them up. And someone will always call others out on their BS.

Whoever is on your team has to be strong and on your side.

Why should you have support around you?

When you lose focus, they will help find it again. As a business owner or a corporate type there are going to be times when you go off track. I know for us when we start getting negative thoughts or getting down on ourselves or feeling lost it's because we have detached ourselves from our purpose from what we're here on this planet to do. We reach out to one of our coaches and tell them how we're feeling. They ask me a couple of questions and bring me right back on track.

In our support network we've currently got:

- *Richard – Business mentor*
- *Ellie – Business mentor & friend*
- *Zoe – Business mentor*
- *Sally – Business mentor/support network*

- *Louise – Spiritual and Emotional mentor*
- *Close friends (especially Kay who helped us with this book)*
- *Family*
- *Clients*

When we need to, we bring in our friends and family for feedback and we also use our clients as well. Our clients give us great feedback because we give no BS to them and they give us the same no BS back.

All of these mentors are professionals we pay for their services. We have got people around us who are at a higher level than us who we look up to and will already have done what we're doing. The big thing here is speed. We could do it on our own but it's probably going to take five, ten, fifteen times the length of time it would do than having these people to ask.

Are you truly connected? Here are the questions we want you to ask yourself today:

- *Am I truly connected to these people?*

____

____

____

____

- *Do I know how to ask for help?*

- *Who are the people who support me?*

- *Who coaches and mentors me?*

- *Who supports my dreams and goals?*

- *Are the people around me equipped to create what I want to create?*

- *Who challenges and pushes me?*

- *Who brings out the best in me?*

- *Who lifts me up?*

- *Who is there to help me grow and develop?*

____

____

____

____

All of these questions relate to any area you want to move your life forward in – whether it's your business or your health or some other area.

In those times when you're feeling hot under the collar or worrying that you aren't good enough, they might help you see what's happening from a different perspective. They can help you to see your strengths and superpowers when you're failing to see them yourself.

We need those people who are going to be really honest with us and call us on it when we're off track or not acting on what we want to achieve. It's great to have people who will sympathise when we're having a bad day but it's just as important to have someone who reminds us that we need to get up tomorrow and get back into it, no excuses.

Sometimes our friends can be the best people to talk to and get support from but sometimes they're not the right people because they're not equipped to advise on how to move forward in our business.

CONCLUSION

Huge congratulations for finishing the book. It's a great achievement to get this far. If you've completed all of the questions, activities and exercises then you will already be able to see the light at the end of the tunnel.

As we finish writing this book, we are so happy. It's been one of our most important goals, to share what we've learned and experienced with more people than we can possibly reach one-to-one. It has felt crazy to keep this stuff to ourselves and only share it with our clients. No matter how many clients we get to, and the numbers are rising every single day, we can't get to everyone.

Burn-out has become a household term because so many people are experiencing it. We don't want everyone to find out how to manage their energy because, like Loz, they hit their big bang and have no choice. Starting from empty will still work, but how much better would it be if we never reached that point.

We do what we do because we love it. Not being able to do it because we have consistently let our own energy cup run dry isn't the ideal approach.

The chances are that you've picked up this book because you are recognising some of the symptoms of burn-out. You may be experiencing symptoms in each of the 3 dimensions of burn-out – physical, mental and emotional.

Our energy reset programme works – it's tried and tested. A word that is not used often enough is 'proven'. We have proven in our own lives that this works. Loz came from rock bottom and is now leading and living her best life, feeling her best and she won't get back to the bottom because she is consistently filling her energy cup. We can't give our best to you, if we don't look after ourselves. But it's not just us – our clients have proven that it works.

You can follow these steps and you will sustainably and simply, in a satisfying way, change your entire life.

We've taken the 3 dimensions of burn-out and applied our 6 pillars of health to them, to give you a more practical understanding and application to them:

Physical/Exhaustion	Sleep
	Water
	Nutrition
	Movement
Mental/Cynicism	Thought management
Emotional/Powerlessness	DeStress/MeTime

We've shared our critical five steps in our energy reset programme for success to keeping that energy cup of yours filled:

1. *The Space*
2. *The Insight*
3. *The Permission*
4. *The Focus*
5. *The Connection*

We do want to remind you at this point that this programme isn't something you can cherry pick. Each of these steps are critical to complete before you move on to the next step or this change will simply not be sustainable. You can stop, BUT if that's what you've always done and you've haven't achieved what you wanted or needed, our suggestion is to try something new – stick with it. Take each step, complete it and THEN move on. You won't regret it.

To make sure it's not overwhelming we've shared with you our 4 'S's ethos of making your changes:

1. *Simple*
2. *Satisfying*
3. *Sustainable*
4. *and within a Supportive community*

If it's not simple and satisfying you won't stick with it, which means it won't be sustainable. AND you don't need to do it by yourself. In fact, we KNOW it's better if you don't. Others who love us and care about our success will support us and keep us accountable.

Don't rush through the 5 steps, take your time. We estimate it will take at least 2 weeks to work through this book.

We've got a free Burn-out Assessment Quiz you can access here to help you get a sense of where you are at. Sometimes it's hard to sit back and assess ourselves, this Quiz will really help. You can find it by scanning this code with your phone camera and clicking on the link

We really, really want you to understand that your motto for success needs to be 'Progress, not perfection'. Perfection isn't possible for any of us so it can't be our goal. Even achieving your ultimate goal in a part of your life will take time but every single step you take towards that goal is progress and worth celebrating. Enough of those steps and you will achieve your goal.

The great news is that while truly changing your energy will take 12 months you will see progress and feel it in your energy levels with every small step you take. You will notice positive differences in a month, much more in 3 months, fantastic change within 6 months and in 12 months you won't believe how filled up your cup is.

Please don't judge yourself harshly as you work through this book and put these simple, satisfying and sustainable changes in place. Judgement is a negative energy. It changes nothing. It's no recipe for success. Be kind to yourself and by default you will find that you will be kinder to others around you.

It goes without saying that if you want us to be your support and you want us to be your support crew through these changes then we would be more than happy to help. This is our jam and we know we can help you.

Our incredibilty popular Energised Leadership Program deals with the three stages of burnout that are affected by your health, mentally, physically and emotionally with the six pillars of health and well-being.

It will enable you to master your energy so you can create

a transformation in your health for which the side effects to your relationships, life, business and career are impactful.

If you would like to explore what it would look like to work together then message us at lauraash@rocksolidhealth.co.uk with the subject line ENERGY RESET BOOK and we can make sure that you get what you need.

WHEEL OF LIFE EXERCISE

First, we want to repeat what we said earlier in the book. We use the Wheel of Life to help our clients see they already have a blueprint of success. Quite often we tend to think we're not successful when we look at something like our health and wellbeing. We think we're completely hopeless and that can become our focus BUT the truth of the matter is that there is a blueprint for success in everything you do. It's about understanding what that blueprint is – then taking it and applying it into other areas of your life.

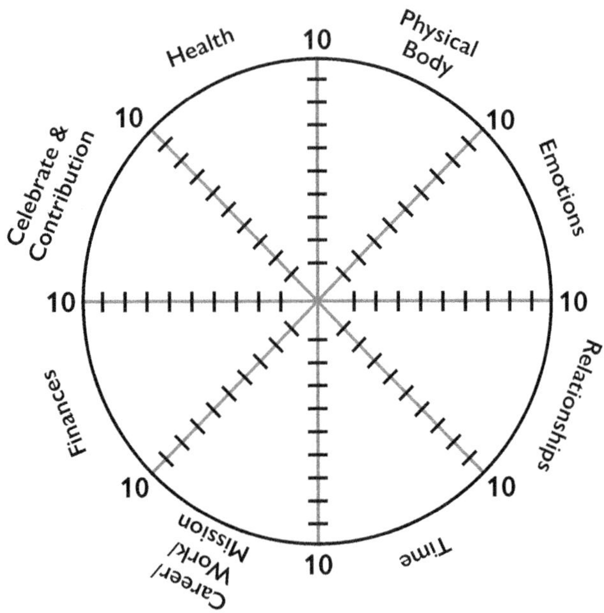

If you look at the Wheel of Life image, there are different areas outlined in it like career, finances, contribution, family relationships, physical body and other parts of your life that are important to you.

What we want you to do is to rate each of those parts from 0 to 10, with zero being the least happy and 10 being amazing. Consider the parts that are somewhere between 8 and 10, often those are the business and career related sections.

Why do you think those areas are scoring so high for you? Consider the following:

- *How much time, work and effort have you invested in these areas?*
- *Have you invested in education or training to achieve those results?*
- *Do you have a clear vision or goal of what you want to achieve in these areas?*
- *Do you feel like you are helping people or making a contribution in what you do for a living?*
- *Do you really enjoy what you're doing?*

Whatever your answers are in the section above, these are the factors that create a blueprint for success. They are a blueprint for an 8-10 result on your Wheel of Life. So, you DO have a blueprint for success and no doubt you can see that for yourself in those areas you are really happy with what you've achieved.

Most often peoples' blueprints for success include 5 main attributes:

- *Dedication*
- *Goals and visions*
- *Learning, study, education*
- *Investing time and effort*
- *Persistence and tenacity*

These factors are the reasons that we have succeeded and achieved in our own lives. All of the parts of our life that we have identified as important to us rate between 8 and 10 because we follow everything we've talked about in this book.

So, let's turn the tables and look at those areas that you've rated as lower on the Wheel of Life. What areas have you chosen 0 to 4? Are they about your physical body, emotions, mental health, relationships? Have a look at your Wheel of Life and note those that are not where you want them to be.

Why do you think they aren't where you want them to be? Consider some of the following:

- *Because of a lack of confidence or self-belief?*
- *No set clear goals or vision?*
- *You haven't invested in yourself?*
- *You haven't invested in learning or support to help you?*

Consider this – what if you approached the areas, you're not happy with, that aren't rating high in your Wheel of Life, the same way you addressed those that are? What if you applied these five pillars to your health, emotions or relationships – or whichever areas you have rated between 0 and 4 on the wheel:

1. *Dedication*
2. *Goals and visions*
3. *Learning, study, education*
4. *Investing time and effort*
5. *Persistence and tenacity*

If you invested time, effort, persistence and learning wouldn't you achieve the same 8 to 10 ratings for those areas? If you set clear goals, wouldn't you get the same outcomes as those areas you are succeeding in?

Using those things that have helped you succeed in the areas you are rating highly in write down why. Then pin that up on the wall, somewhere you can see it every day. Whenever you think about your health, your physical body, your mental health think about it from that blueprint. Think about how you can apply those to the areas you want to improve on. It's a great reminder of the areas you're successful in which will motivate you and help to think about how easily you could transfer that success to other parts of your life that are important to you.

If you do the Wheel of Life 3months, 6months or 12 months after you've transferred that successful formula over to those other areas in your life, you'll see how much you've achieved. You will see for yourself that you DO have a blueprint for success.

WHERE YOUR FOCUS GOES, YOUR ENERGY FLOWS AND YOUR ACHIEVEMENTS GROW.

ACKNOWLEDGEMENTS

We want to thank every one of our clients, mentors, coaches, friends, family members, colleagues past and present, and those who we are yet to meet, for helping us grow, learn and become who we are today and who we will become.

If it was not for you then we would not have the courage, skills, talents or abilities to be able to make this book a reality and be of service, so that we can simply leave this earth in a better state than how we found it.

Energy Reset: Powerfully align your energy to create more abundance in your business, career, health and life

Please can we give a huge thank you to you Danny Lyle for helping us design the book!!!

ENDNOTES

1 https://www.who.int/news/item/28-05-2019-burn-out-an-occupational-phenomenon-international-classification-of-diseases
2 https://dictionary.cambridge.org/dictionary/english/burn-out
3 https://www.ncbi.nlm.nih.gov/pmc/articles/PMC4525425/
4 https://www.ncbi.nlm.nih.gov/pmc/articles/PMC6305886/)
5 https://dictionary.cambridge.org/dictionary/english/connection

Printed in Great Britain
by Amazon

38500623R00126